Communication Skills for Nursing Practice

Catherine McCabe
Fiona Timmins

Consultant editor: Jo Campling

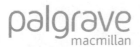

palgrave
macmillan

First published 2006 by
PALGRAVE MACMILLAN
Houndmills, Basingstoke, Hampshire RG21 6XS and
175 Fifth Avenue, New York, N.Y. 10010
Companies and representatives throughout the world

PALGRAVE MACMILLAN is the global academic imprint of the
Palgrave Macmillan division of St. Martin's Press, LLC and of
Palgrave Macmillan Ltd. Macmillan® is a registered trademark in
the United States, United Kingdom and other countries. Palgrave is
a registered trademark in the European Union and other countries.

ISBN-13: 978 1 4039 4985 1
ISBN 10: 1 4039 4985 9

This book is printed on paper suitable for recycling and
made from fully managed and sustained forest sources.

A catalogue record for this book is available from the British
Library.

10   9   8   7   6   5   4   3   2   1
16   15   14   13   12   11   10   09   08   07

Printed and bound in China

To Kevin, Jessica, Niamh and Andrew
To Bernard, Kerry-Anne and Nathan

·

Contents

List of figures

Acknowledgements

We would like to thank Professor Cecily Begley, Vice Dean, Faculty of Health Sciences, University of Dublin, Trinity College Dublin, for her support an encouragement throughout the preparation of this book. We are also grateful to the staff at Palgrave Macmillan for their invaluable support. Finally we are indebted to Jo Campling for her contribution towards both the conception and completion of this book.

Every effort has been made to trace all copyright holders but if any have been inadvertently overlooked the publishers will be pleased to make the necessary arrangement at the first opportunity.

PART I

The theoretical foundations of
communication in nursing

1 Communication theory

Introduction

Communication is something that we all do whether we want to or not, even if we hide ourselves away and cannot be seen, we are still communicating that we are unhappy or do not wish to see other people. We cannot prevent ourselves from communicating, even if we try not to speak to someone, our bodies will betray us and send a message to the other person. So we are all compelled to communicate at some level by using language and our bodies. However, communication does not always seem to work effectively. Why is this? Why do we walk away from encounters feeling angry, humiliated, frustrated and thinking to ourselves, 'if only I had said . . .' On the other hand why do we walk away from situations leaving others feeling like this? Indeed, how often are we actually aware that our communication has possibly engendered negative feelings in others?

Exercise

To what extent are you aware of the impact of your communication behaviours on others? You should write down your thoughts on this before proceeding with the chapter.

It could be argued that communication is not actually communication unless it is intentional. In other words if you are angry about losing a purse/wallet and this is evident in your facial expression and tone when you are speaking to someone else about an unrelated matter, then it doesn't count as relevant to the interaction. This may be the case

3

from your perspective but when communicating, you need to consider and be aware of the effect your facial expression and tone has on another person. Your behaviour whether verbal or non-verbal, will influence how another person communicates with you because of the message that body language sends out.

This book is concerned with interpersonal communication in nursing, regardless of the medium through which it takes place. The emphasis is on the verbal and/or non-verbal language required to deliver the message in a manner that is patient-centred, respectful, genuine and therapeutic. This requires a level of awareness, not just of the specific nature and purpose of the message but most importantly it requires a knowledge of ones self. Communication is about interacting with people and, therefore, is at the core of nursing. For nursing care to be effective and therapeutic, the communication skills used by nurses need to be patient-centred. This requires a continuing awareness by nurses as individuals of their contribution to interactions that they have not just with patients but also with relatives, friends, other health care professionals and health care staff. Nurses often find it difficult to define their role but nonetheless it is clear that nurses spend more time with patients than any other health care professional and co-ordinate their care by communicating closely with these other professionals. Without attempting to define all aspects of nursing, communication is without doubt an integral part of the nurse's role.

Concepts of communication

This chapter will examine communication as a concept; first, by exploring non-nursing communication models that we frequently refer to when we think or learn about communication. Second, in order to consider communication in a context that we believe is unique to nursing, we will then look at models of communication specific to the nurse's role.

Communication has been described as being both a simple and a complex process (Rosengren, 2000). The Linear Model of Communication (Miller and Nicholson, 1976) may be

Exercise

Here is a question for you and one that you may not have considered previously, 'What is Communication'? Try to write down the first ideas that come into your head and keep them close by, as you will need to refer back to them as you read on.

considered as an illustration of simple communication. This is illustrated as follows:

Sender → Message → Receiver

Berlo (1960) and Miller and Nicholson (1976) described communication as, quite simply, an activity. In this activity, a sender transmits a message to a receiver in order to bring about a desired response. Communication is said to occur in one direction only. The sender is responsible for not only the accuracy of the content but also the tone of the message. The message contains verbal and/or non-verbal information that will be interpreted by the receiver. The sender of the message will know that the receiver has interpreted the message accurately through feedback.

However, based on this model, for communication to be effective it is assumed that the sender is very clear about the purpose of the message and what it is supposed to achieve and has also carefully considered the recipient when formulating the message. It is also assumed with this model that the recipient is an open-minded and willing participant in the interaction. These assumptions do not take into account other factors (intrinsic and extrinsic) that can influence the communication process. Intrinsic factors apply to both the sender and receiver and refer to personal and professional aspects of a person that may affect communication. Examples of these are values, beliefs, culture, goals, role and knowledge/education in relation to the topic of communication. Extrinsic factors that may influence the communication process relate to the immediate physical environment and the communication medium being used. DeVito (2002) described these factors as 'noise' that could distort the message being transmitted and distort the perception of the receiver, such that the message is interpreted differently to the original meaning intended by the sender. DeVito (2002) described four types of noise;

1 Physical noise (external to the speaker, for example, Loud music or voices in the background);
2 Physiological noise (physical impairments that influence perception by the receiver);
3 Psychological noise (perceptions of sender/receiver being influenced by individual beliefs, values, biases, goals); and
4 Semantic noise (words have different meanings in different contexts)

The linear model of communication is, therefore, limited and perhaps is most useful for identifying the basic components of simple communication, rather than for illustrating the complexities of communication between humans.

The Circular Transactional Model of Communication, based on the work of Bateson (1979) takes a broader view of the communication process (Figure 1.1). Communication comprises similar components as the linear model but the concept of communication is further developed by the indication that all communication is interpersonal, therefore, it takes place within the context of a relationship. This model acknowledged the key role that intrinsic and extrinsic factors outlined above or 'noise' play in the communication process, but it also included the concepts of 'feedback' and 'validation' as fundamental for the development and continuation of successful or effective communication.

Both of these concepts will be discussed in Chapter 3 in relation to therapeutic communication. The transactional nature of this model lies in its recognition of communication as a reciprocal process in which communication is simultaneous and shared between people as 'communicators' rather than a 'sender' and 'receiver'. The cyclical aspect of this model acknowledged that communication is not linear or one-way but is instead an ongoing dynamic process that is inherently complex.

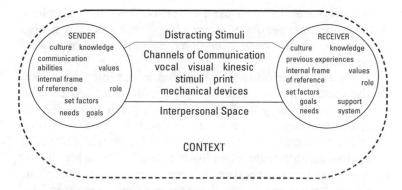

Source: Arnold, E. and Boggs, K. (1995) *Interpersonal Relationships: Professional Communication Skills for Nurses*, 2nd edn. Reproduced with permission from Elsevier Inc.

Figure 1.1 Picture of circular transactional model of communication

Hargie and Dickson (2004) developed another model of communication entitled 'A Skill Model of Interpersonal Communication'. It contains many of the elements illustrated in the circular transaction model of communication but presented these elements as skills, suggesting that effective or successful interpersonal communication is purposeful and focused. These skills are identified as follows:

- person-situation context;
- goal;
- mediating processes;
- response;
- feedback; and
- perception.

The person-situation context refers to the individual or unique aspects of a person that contribute to an interaction. These aspects include the person's values, beliefs, culture, knowledge, skills, personality, age, gender, self-concept and self-efficacy (self-belief in one's ability to succeed) and may influence their approach and style of response during an interaction. The situation itself in terms of not just the physical setting but the parameters (roles and rules) will also directly impact on how people behave and respond during an interaction.

The goal of the individuals involved in the interaction may be the same or it may differ to a greater or lesser degree. The achievement of the goal influences each participant's behaviour, and persistence, appropriateness and selectivity are three behaviours described by Oettingen and Gollwitzer (2001) as evident when in pursuit of individual goals. The achievement of goals depends on whether the goals are implicit or explicit, how important they are, whether they are task- or relationship-related, how compatible the goals of the people are and whether they are primary or secondary goals.

Mediating processes refer to a combination of cognitive and affective processes that help the participants in the interaction to work through the encounter by identifying goals and acknowledging and responding to events. Cognitive processes are concerned with how individuals have a very personal way of using their knowledge and beliefs when thinking about things and this directly impacts on how they problem-solve, make judgements or perceive situations generally. The affective process is based on an individual's value system and the way in which it influences our attitude towards our actions and interactions with others. A crucial aspect of mediating processes is that a tentative or flexible outcome (strategy or plan for achieving a goal) is reached.

The 'responses' aspect of the skills model relates to the implementation of the agreed strategy or plan. Responses incorporate the use of verbal and non-verbal communication, which along with environmental and organizational factors can influence the smooth or bumpy implementation of the strategy or plan.

Feedback is described by Hargie and Dickson (2004) as an integral ingredient in the communication process. Feedback lets everyone in the interaction know that the message has been received and also lets the sender know how those who received it have interpreted it. Feedback is evident from both verbal and non-verbal responses equally and clarifies whether interpretation or understanding of the message is mutual or shared. This allows the communication to continue and strategies and plans to be refined and implemented.

Perception refers to the way we perceive others and the context in which an interaction takes place is the primary influence on what happens in the interaction and also what the outcome of the interaction is. According to Hargie and Dickson (2004), in order to predict how an interaction will proceed and its outcome, we need to be aware of and monitor ourselves in terms of our performance and contribution to the interaction and that failure to do this may result in regular experiences of ineffective communication or unwanted outcomes from interactions.

Defining communication

It is difficult to define communication and looking at these models presented it is easy to see why. The linear model represents only one minor aspect of communication and that is communication that is one directional and does not recognize the influence of the individual or the environment in the communication process and the complexities therein. The circular transactional model is broader in that it recognizes the influence that the individual and the context have on the communication process and the importance of feedback and validation in allowing the interaction to be interpreted and expected outcome to be agreed. The skills model of interpersonal communication is based on similar components but includes key ingredients such as the goal of the interaction, individual perceptions and the mediating processes that play a fundamental role in the development and outcome of an interaction. This model introduces the notion that communication requires certain skills in order to be successful for all those involved in the interaction. So it could be said that communication is not a simple process in any interaction or situation and to regard it as such would require that the dynamic individual and contextual nature of communication be ignored or underestimated.

Let's look at the various definitions of communication that are provided by some authors on the topic:

Interpersonal communication can be thought of as a process that is transactional, purposeful, multi-dimensional, irreversible and (possibly) inevitable. (Hargie and Dickson, 2004, p. 41)

Interpersonal skills are Goal-directed behaviours used in face-to-face interactions, which are effective in bringing about a desired state of affairs. (Hayes, 1991, p. 5)

Communication involves the reciprocal process in which messages are sent and received between two or more people. (Balzer-Riley, 2004, p. 6)

A useful way of thinking about interpersonal communication is as a series of messages – information – which you send out to other people and messages which you received from them, through seeing, hearing or touching one another. (Petrie, 1997, p. 6)

Communication is a universal function of man that is not tied to any particular place, time or context. (Ruesch, 1961, pp. 30–1)

The diversity of these definitions in terms of their broadness or even vagueness highlights the complexity of the concept of communication and, therefore, the difficulty in producing a comprehensive model and definition of communication that truly reflects its essence. The definitions supplied by Balzer-Riley (2004), Hargie and Dickson (2004), Hayes (1991) and Petrie (1997) all used terms such as 'interpersonal communication' and 'interpersonal skills' interchangeably and are based on the fundamental belief that communication is an interpersonal process. Ruesch (1961) did not concur with this view. His definition described communication as a function, which implied that it is always purposeful. However, none of these definitions or models provides possible explanations as to why some communication is positive and some is not. Take a look at the following interaction:

Smiling and in a friendly tone, a nurse asks her nursing colleague, 'Are you free to check the medication with me now?' Her colleague is reading some notes and she looks and sounds irritated when she replies, 'Yes, OK but it will have to be quick; the new admission will be here in fifteen minutes.' The first nurse seems confused by this reaction and says 'If you are busy I will ask someone else . . .' Her colleague immediately says 'No, no, I'm sorry if I seem irritable, its just that I was looking at the duty roster and I am working on my birthday.'

This type of interaction is quite common between colleagues or friends and is an example of both intrapersonal and interpersonal communication. The colleague probably did look irritated but this was due to her own private thoughts in relation to having to work on her birthday and her face registered these inner feelings. However, the first nurse perceived the irritated expression as being directed at her. The problem is that often an individual's intrapersonal communication is evident in their facial expression and a message is sent to the outside and is observed and interpreted by other people but this message is not, nor was never intended to be, a message to another person. This is an example of unconscious communication that can have a negative effect on an interaction. The nurses communicated well in this example and nobody was left feeling negative about the interaction but often such inter actions can cause friction and bad feeling among colleagues. Of course, the opposite is also possible, that is, communication that is successful and has a positive outcome can also be the result of communication that is unconscious.

Mindful of this and in view of the models of communication reviewed we propose that communication is probably best described as a complex, unconscious or deliberate process

Exercise

Previously in this chapter you were asked to consider what you think communication is and write it down. Now having read about some communication models and definitions have a look at what you have written and decide whether you want to make any adjustments. When you are happy with this, answer these questions:

● What is communication in nursing?
● Is it different to communication in the other health care professionals?

Again, write down the thoughts that come into your head and keep them, as you will need to refer to them again when you have finished this chapter and others in this book.

that influences the development of interpersonal or professional relationships and outcomes of interactions, regardless of the context.

We regard communication in nursing as different to communication in the other health care professionals. It is unique, not because of the communication skills required, since any professional working with the public needs to have effective communications skills, but rather because of the focus and emphasis of communication in the professional practice of nursing. Nurses are at the coal-face of the health care services. They spend more time with patients than perhaps any other health care professionals. The focus of this time is often on co-ordinating, explaining and delivering patient care using therapeutic communication. The emphasis of this time is (or should be) facilitating individual patient's needs. It is widely recognized that communication is practically unavoidable and is to do with people interacting and developing relationships and working and living together. Therefore, it follows that as nursing is about helping people, the communication of information and feelings between the nurse and the patient and the nurse and other health care professionals is an integral part of how nurses do their job. Authors such as Attree (2001), Fosbinder (1994), Peplau (1988), Sheppard (1993), Thorsteinsson (2002) and Wilkinson (1999) support this view and also suggest that the development of a positive nurse–patient relationship is essential for the delivery of high quality nursing care.

Models of communication in nursing

Previously in this chapter we looked at three models of communication. It became evident that the linear model, which depicts one-way communication, is limited in its application and not congruent with the multidimensional nature of communication in nursing. The circular transactional model and the skills model of interpersonal communication are certainly more useful in explaining the processes and components of interpersonal communication required in nursing.

There are very few models of communication that relate to

specifically to nursing, however, authors such as Fosbinder (1994) and Morse *et al.* (1992) and Morse *et al.* (1997) have made significant contributions to this aspect of nursing. In her study, Fosbinder (1994) asked patients to describe what happened when the nurse was taking care of them. The inter-personal competence of the nurse was the primary concern of the patients and four interpersonal processes emerged from what they described. These were:

- translating;
- getting to know you;
- establishing trust; and
- going the extra mile.

The key components of translating include information giving, explaining and instructing. Getting to know you relates to being friendly, using humour in interactions and personal sharing. Establishing trust relates to the confidence that patients have in the nurse's professional competence and demeanour. It requires that nurses anticipate patient needs, follow through and appear to enjoy the job. The last process, going the extra mile, relates to being a friend and doing more for the patient than is required. This is not something that patients expect from every nurse but it is described as a special, less-formal relationship between a nurse and patient. As you can see the main focus of these four processes is interpersonal competence and communication and if you consider the components of each of these processes, the communication skills required are not highly specialized, most of us could achieve them without even realizing it. What makes this model so important and relevant is that its content is derived directly from patients and, therefore, provides key information to nurses about how patients want them to communicate.

Morse *et al.* (1992) developed a model of communication that focused on the emotional engagement of the nurse with the patient (Figure 1.2). The model is based on two key characteristics. The first is whether the nurse is patient-focused or nurse-focused and the second is whether the communication is spontaneous (first-level) or learned (second-level). The patient-focused, first-level communication is emotionally

FOCUS

	Sufferer-focused (patient)		Self-focused (professional)	
	CHARACTERISTIC	RESPONSE	RESPONSE	CHARACTERISTIC
First-level	Engaged (with sufferer's emotion) Genuine Reflexive	Pity Sympathy Consolation Commiseration Compassion Reflexive reassurance	Guarding Shielding/steeling/ bracing Dehumanizing Withdrawing Distancing Labelling Denying	Anti-engaged (against embodiment; protective)
Second-level	Pseudo-engaged Learned Professional	Sharing self Humour Reassurance (informing) Therapeutic empathy Confronting Comforting (learned)	Rote behaviours 'professional style' Legitimizing/ justifying Pity (false/ professional) Stranger Reassurance (false)	A-engaged (embodiment absent or removed)

Source: Morse, J.M., Bottorff, J., Anderson, G., O'Brien, B. and Solberg, S. (1992) Beyond empathy: Expanding expressions of caring, *Journal of Advanced Nursing*, 17, 809–21, with permission from Blackwell Publishing.

Figure 1.2   Model of communication

driven and culturally conditioned and, therefore, it is often an unconscious response. This type of communication includes responses such as pity, sympathy, consolation, compassion, commiseration and reflexive reassurance, which we would often regard as normal every day communication but which is often undervalued and regarded as superficial (McQueen, 2002; Morse *et al.* 1992). Sympathy, for example, which Morse *et al.* (1992, p. 812) define as 'an expression of the caregiver's own sorrow at another's plight' can make patients feel understood and comforted because the nurse has recognized how unwell they may be feeling. This narrative from a study on nurse–patient communication by McCabe (2004, p. 45) illustrates this point: 'I liked them [nurses] all, but there was one little girl, she was slightly different – sympathetic I would say. I think the patient deserves sympathy when they are hospitalized, their complaint may not warrant sympathy but they're away from their own environment . . .' (Sophie)

Patient-focused, second-level (learned) communication includes responses such as sharing self, confronting, comforting, humour and informative reassurance. These responses may be difficult for some nurses at under-graduate level because although they may argue that they are using humour and sharing self with their patients, they need to consider carefully whether this type of interaction is patient-focused or whether it is focused on themselves. Talking about their personal and social lives and using humour is important in helping students to relax and establish relationships with patients. Often, patients enjoy these interactions too, which may help to alleviate the boredom of hospital life. However, nursing students need to be mindful as they try to develop their confidence and communication skills, that the focus of interactions with patients should always be the patient. This does not mean that you should not talk about yourself, in fact, when you first meet a patient, it is often necessary to talk about yourself first in order to make the patient feel comfortable. Talking to a patient about where you come from, your family and even your social life may seem like a social conversation and, therefore, perhaps not that important. However it provides the nurse with the opportunity to ask the patient about himself or herself and helps the nurse to establish a rapport with the patient and try to determine what their needs are. For the patient this type of conversation gives them the opportunity to decide if the nurse is a good person and if they trust them or not and it also provides normal social interactions that patients often miss when they are in hospital.

Nurse-focused, first-level responses include guarding, dehumanizing, withdrawing, distancing, labelling and denying, often delivered using the busy nurse persona. These can be conscious or unconscious responses that nurses use to detach from difficult or emotional situations in an effort to overcome stress or very intense feelings. The difficulty with this type of communication is that it can be over-used because it allows nurses to get their work done with minimal emotional distraction; however it can result in isolating patients and making them feel anxious and lonely.

Nurse-focused, second-level communication includes rote or mechanical responses, false pity and false reassurance.

Nurses who communicate in this way can appear distant and uncaring to their patients and this can make patients feel under-valued as individuals. This lowers their self-esteem and may prevent them from trusting the nurses and talking to the nurses about how they are feeling, either physically or psychologically. As nurses, phrases like 'Don't worry' and 'Everything will be fine' tend to come easily but they fall under the heading of the nurse-focused, second-level communication or false-reassurance even if they are spoken with the best of intentions. Statements like these to patients can make them feel that they are over-reacting to their own illness or possibly that nobody is interested in their worries or fears. Nurses may use these responses uncon-sciously to prevent the patient from verbalizing any further fears. This is because the emotions that are evident in the patient are those that the nurse may start to feel are too difficult or intense to deal with, or they may feel that they do not have time to listen and then deal with the issues that the patient raises.

The model of communication developed by Morse *et al.* (1992) (Figure 1.2) is quite a comprehensive model as it relates across many nursing contexts and disciplines. For example, it is applicable in areas like day surgery or emergency nursing where the nurse–patient relationship is transient and its duration is limited. It is also relevant in areas where the nurse–patient relationship is long-term, for example long-stay units, residential homes or when caring for chronically or terminally ill patients. This model is particularly useful for helping nurses identify communication responses that consti-tute patient-focused communication and those that constitute nurse-focused communication. As previously mentioned, patient-focused, first level emotion-based responses such as pity, sympathy and compassion are often undervalued in nurs-ing whereas concepts that offer a detached, more controlling approach to communication such as therapeutic empathy and counselling are often referred to as essential communication skills for nurses. These skills are derived from counselling theory, they require specific skills to be used by counsellors in very controlled atmospheres and focus on facilitating clients to come up with solutions for their problems. These concepts will be developed further in Chapter 4 when we talk about helping skills and empathy.

Morse *et al.* (1997) devised 'The Comforting Interaction-Relationship Model' which is based on nurse–patient interaction as a strategy for the nurse and the patient to establish a therapeutic relationship through negotiation. This model proposed that the primary goal of nursing is to help patients reach an acceptable comfort level while receiving essential nursing care. The model reflects aspects of the circular transactional model and the skills model of communication and it is an important model for nurses because it is patient-centred and recognizes that nurse–patient interactions and relationships are dynamic and should be interactive and guided by the context in which they occur. This model utilizes Peplau's (1952, p. 9) definition of 'relationship' as 'two persons come to know each other well enough to face the problems at hand in a co-operative way'. This means that even very short-duration nurse–patient interactions can be regarded as relationships even though the nurse and patient may have only just met. Morse *et al.* (1997) identified three components to the model: nursing actions; patient actions; and the evolving relationship.

Nursing actions occur simultaneously, are interactive and consist of:

- *Comforting strategies* such as touch and listening that can be planned or subconscious, direct or indirect actions but to be successful they must be patient-centred, i.e. used in response to a patient cue. An example of this is if a patient winces because they are in pain, then the nurse speaks softly and uses gentle touch.
- *Styles of care*, which relates the use of a combination of particular comfort strategies.
- *Nursing patterns of relating* are learned professional behaviours using a combination of styles of care. As nurses become socialized and gain more experience, they use standardized and normative patterns of relating. These patterns vary depending on the nursing specialty and the nurses' role, for example, nurses working in emergency departments will use a different way of relating and behaving to nurses working in community care.

Patient actions consist of:

- *Signals of discomfort*, which can be verbal, non-verbal, situational or environmental, for example, a patient may state that they are experiencing pain or they may indicate by constantly shifting in the bed that they are in pain or they find it difficult to sleep because of noise around them during the day or night.
- *Indices of distress* emerge from signals of discomfort that a patient may give and they indicate that the patient needs a nursing intervention, for example, pre-operatively a patient may appear agitated, restless, wringing their hands. By talking to the patient and reassuring them, the nurse can reduce the patient's level of stress.
- *Patterns of relating to a nurse* are only developed when a patient decides whether or not they trust the nurse, and relinquishes to care or rejects nursing interventions. At this stage in the relationship, the patient controls the response of the nurse and the nature of the subsequent relationship. This means that this model recognizes that the patient has ultimate control in the type of relationship that develops between the nurse and patient.

The *evolving relationship* is the third component of this model and it describes nursing and patient actions as the means by which the nurse–patient relationship is negotiated and subsequently develops. Nurses respond to patient signals of discomfort and indices of distress using comforting strategies, styles of caring and patterns of relating on an ongoing and changing basis.

One important aspect to nurse–patient communication, and you may have noticed this already, is its 'unconscious' nature. Often our communication with others is unconscious, i.e. we have many interactions with people but often we are unaware of our personal contribution to the interaction. How then can nurses be certain that the way they communicate is patient-centred? Bradley and Edinberg (1990) and Kruijver *et al.* (2001) suggested that nurses regularly use the linear model of one-way communication when caring for patients and the reasons for this have already been alluded to.

These are that they often profess to be too busy to deal with the unexpected and possibly difficult concerns that patients may have or they may also feel that they just do not have the time to actually listen. One-way communication allows nurses to control the interaction and when nurses feel that they have a lot of work to do or tasks to complete, this is a useful way of communicating. However, the consequence of this type of communication is that it does not recognize the patient as the centre of care but rather the nurse's need to complete the task takes precedence over the needs of the patient. Interestingly Astedt-Kurki and Haggman-Laitila (1992) and Williams (1998) argue that patient-centred communication does not necessarily take up more of the nurse's time, it is not, they suggested, an additional task for the nurse. Rather it is simply portrayed by nurses in the words and body language that they choose to use when approaching patients. This notion, and its relationship to the concept of patient-centred communication forms the basis of Morse *et al.*'s (1997) model and will be discussed in greater detail in Chapter 3.

 Exercise

Before you read the next chapter ask yourself the following questions:

- In what situations am I most aware of how I communicate at work?
- In what situations am I most aware of how I communicate in my personal life?
- Are these situations where I am striving to meet my own needs?

When you have written down your answers read them back and ascertain whether or nor they reflect a patient-centred approach to care.

Key points

▶ We communicate because as human beings, we are compelled to.

▶ The way we, as individuals, communicate influences the type of relationship we have with others.

▶ Communication in nursing is concerned with providing individualized nursing care and co-ordinating interdisciplinary care in a patient-centred way.

▶ Communication is a complex, dynamic process that often occurs outside a person's awareness.

▶ In order for communication to be effective and patient-centred, nurses need to develop awareness of how they communicate and the influence this has on the nurse–patient relationship.

▶ Good communication is not more time consuming than bad communication.

2 Nursing theory

Introduction

Securing and practicing from a uniform knowledge base is essential to the development of the discipline of nursing. Nursing theory has not only the potential to inform nursing practice, but also allows empirical examination of nursing interventions. Nursing theory has a great deal to contribute to our knowledge and understanding of communication and in this chapter we examine theories of nursing and outline how they may be used in nursing practice to enhance nurse–patient communication. This knowledge of specific nursing theory will help to build upon definitions of communication developed in the previous chapter. The understanding of communication will broaden to encompass nursing's unique role and function in this domain as outlined by various theorists.

Although the nursing theories presented have unique foci upon nursing care, their emphasis on communication within the health care setting and the nurse–patient relationship is common to all. There is a common belief among theorists that communication within a nurse–patient relationship is a fundamental aspect of nursing care delivery. We intend to impart the importance of communication and discuss the relevance of views of communication and the impact that this may have on patient outcome.

Barriers to the development of the nurse–patient relationship

One of the fundamental values that should underpin today's nursing practice is the development of a therapeutic relationship between nurse and patient (Arnold and Undermann Boggs, 1999). This relationship is emphasized throughout the literature on the topic (Aggleton and Chalmers, 2000; Howard-Harwood, 1997).

It is only through good communication, and the development of the therapeutic relationship that nurses can truly identify the unique needs of their patients. This process underpins contemporary approaches to information giving and education within the hospital settings (Ito and Lambert, 2002) and supports a nurse–patient communication that is patient centred.

These are barriers to using this approach at a practice level. These concern the failure to individualize nursing care, ritualistic nursing actions and lack of communication skills.

Exercise

Spend some time identifying what you perceive as barriers to the development of the nurse–patient relationship

---

Failure to individualize nursing care

A predominant theme in Costa's (2001) phenomenological study of 16 patients who had undergone day surgery was ' not being recognized as individuals'. Respondents in this study recognized the presence of the nurse as valuable to their recovery, thus indicating the therapeutic potential of the nurse's role itself. Costa (2001) recommended that nurses needed to develop specific therapeutic communication skills including being 'truly present' to the patient. This is manifested by being able to listen, being perceptive to the environment and being able to anticipate patients' needs.

Exercise

Have you noticed occasions where individualized nursing care did not occur? Can you identify possible reasons for this?

Ritualistic nursing actions

Nursing has long been associated with the use of rituals and tradition, and although these have declined in many areas of nursing they still prevail (Jacobson, 2000; Riegel *et al.*, 1996; Strange, 2001). There are a variety of reasons for this; lack of autonomy, lack of knowledge, hierarchical systems and avoidance measures, to name but a few.

This use of rituals affects the nurse's ability to communicate effectively (Martin, 1998). Rather than an open communication system, Martin (1998) suggested that communication rituals are socially constructed within the healthcare setting, and communication during nursing procedures is often condensed and restricted and ultimately a source of patient control, rather than a therapeutic intervention. Furthermore, this ritualistic communication is 'full of jargon and abbreviations impossible for those outside the profession to understand' (Martin, 1998). Little consensus exists regarding the exact origin of ritual within nursing; however, there is consensus that nursing needs to move away from these traditional operating frameworks.

Martin (1998) attributed nurses' use of rituals to what he termed ' professional distancing', whereby, perhaps due to the emotional burden of care, nurses distance themselves from the patients. This distancing has obvious repercussions for nurse–patient communication. The nature of ritualistic communication is unlikely to be patient-centred as it serves the purpose of the nurse. Rituals, Martin (1998) proposed, were also bound in 'task orientation'. Despite a rhetoric of patient-centred care, the focus of many hospital wards is on getting the work done (Martin, 1998). He suggests that this 'contributes to the "busy nurse" syndrome which keeps the nurse active all the time and protects him/her from the need to talk to the patient'. This busyness allows the nurse to 'legitimately distance themselves from patients' thus allowing 'no time for nurse–patient interaction' (Martin, 1998). This has obvious potential repercussions for nurse–patient communication.

This was also evident in Jenner's (1998) case study analysis of nurses' roles, education and training needs associated with patient-focused care. One emerging theme was 'the task skills approach to nurses' competence and the delivery of care'. This theme revealed that the nurses in the study (23) perceived that their preparatory nurse education programme had prepared them mostly for specific skills and duties. 'Task orientation' emerged as a sub-theme. Jenner (1998) attributed this to a coping strategy by nurses.

 Exercise

List and identify nursing rituals that you may have encountered. Can you identify possible reasons for these?

Lack of communication skills

Keating *et al.* (2002) identified barriers to nurse–patient relationships among 119 nurses in Australia. Communication was identified as the principal barrier to the development of the relationship.

While education can have a positive effect on the communication skills of nurses (Chambers-Evans *et al.*, 1999), the lack of good communication skills considered in light of other barriers to the therapeutic relationship (ritualistic nursing actions and failure to individualize nursing care) suggest the need for a holistic framework to guide and direct nursing practice in this area. From a systematic review of the literature Michie *et al.* (2003) identified 'the ability to elicit and discuss patients' beliefs' and ' the ability to activate the patient to take control' as integral components of patient-centred care. Similarly, Fossum and Arborelius (2004) found from an observation study of outpatient doctor–patient interactions that 'involving the patient in management' led to more successful interactions. Fossum and Arborelius (2004) also amalgamated the findings of previous studies into suggestions to improve patient-centred communication. These recommendations included:

● providing the opportunity for the patient to express their needs, including symptoms, thoughts, feelings and expectations;

● treating the patient as a person with a health need, rather than the perception of the person as a disease entity; and
● enabling that the patient to feel that they have been understood.

Patient-centred communication is not only good for patients it is also good for the health care system. Wissow (2004) noted that studies in the USA that compared doctors' malpractice claim histories with their communication skills, found patient-centred practices evident in those with less claims who did more to facilitate patient participation and used more humour, and they advocated its use among doctors.

Patient-centredness requires recognition of the uniqueness of the individual; it requires core communication skills and individual patient needs assessment. These items are central components of nursing theory and the conceptual model used in nursing. Therefore, we will examine theories of nursing and outline how they may be used in nursing practice to enhance nurse–patient communication and the therapeutic relationship, by fostering holistic nursing care. This knowledge of specific nursing theory will help to build upon definitions of communication developed in the previous chapter.

 Exercise

List ways that that you may enhance therapeutic relationships with patients.

What is nursing theory?

One prime motivator for the development of nursing theory in recent decades is the belief that although nurses work in parallel with many other health care professionals, they assess, plan, implement and evaluate care in their own right. They use nursing theory – a suitable theoretical framework with which to conceptualize, describe and inform the unique contribution of the nurse in health care settings – to guide this process.

The complexity of contemporary nursing practice requires a systematic approach that complies with current trends of patient-centred care. Application of nursing theory to practice serves to clarify the nurse's function in nursing situations and provides a rationale for nursing actions. It also offers an unique perspective of the patient that is holistic and not disease focused. Conceptual model use prescribes a systematic approach to care based on sound theoretical principles, with particular emphasis on assessment, planning, implementing and evaluation of care.

The terms 'conceptual models' and 'theory' are often used interchangeably, and while many theorists outline both a theory and a conceptual model, significant differences exist in the definition and understanding of both (Fawcett, 1995). Practicing nurses are most familiar with the use of conceptual models. These are but one component of what Fawcett (1995) referred to as a structural hierarchy of knowledge in nursing (Figure 2.1). The most abstract level of knowledge in the hierarchy being the metaparadigm. This identifies over-arching concepts under consideration. In nursing, these are the person, the environment, health and nursing (Alligood and Marriner-Tomey, 2002a). The metaparadigm doesn't

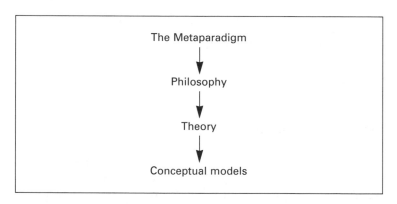

Source: Adapted from Fawcett, J. (1995) *Analysis and Evaluation of Conceptual Models of Nursing* (3rd edition) Philadelphia, F.A. Davies Company.

Figure 2.1 The nursing knowledge hierarchy

provide direct guidance to practice, but rather presents a broad view of the uniform understandings within a discipline that inform the theory.

Philosophy, another component in the hierarchy, is a statement of beliefs (Kim, 1983). Each theory of nursing has its own philosophy that informs the theory. The theory itself, although abstract, guides and informs nursing practice. Conceptual models of nursing represent the final aspect of the knowledge hierarchy. They provide frameworks to guide and direct nursing care. Each conceptual model provides an unique direction to nursing practice (Fawcett, 1995).

Exercise

What does nursing theory mean to you?

The potential contribution of nursing theory to guide communication practice in nursing

Nursing as an unique function outside of medicine is a predominant theme in the literature. The 'medical model' as it is often termed, is the predominant paradigm in many areas of medical practice, where doctors are concerned mainly with disease processes and cure. McKenna (1997) and Pearson *et al.* (2000) argued that while this approach is relevant to medicine, it is not entirely relevant to nursing. Rather than nurses considering patients in terms of their condition or treatment such as 'a hysterectomy', these authors suggested a more holistic, caring approach consistent with the goals of the nursing profession. Nursing theory use facilitates this.

The emergence and continued development of nursing theory and conceptual models to guide practice, which occurred mostly in the USA, has become synonymous with the individualization of patient care. It also serves to reduce the use of ritual, routine, task orientation and use of the medical model through the promotion of thoughtful, insightful care planning for each individual patient (Alligood, 2002).

Nursing theory offers nursing a distinct scientific knowledge base to guide practice. Without the use of nursing theory to guide practice, rituals are likely to prevail. Although there have been and continue to be issues with nursing theory and conceptual model use such as difficulty with relevance and application to practice, concerns about empirical testing and associated documentation, their overall contribution to the individualization of nursing is something that cannot be ignored in a consideration of factors that could improve the nurse–patient therapeutic relationship. In addition, as most nursing theory focuses on communication as a distinct aspect of the role of the nurse, it is important to explore the potential contribution of nursing theory and conceptual models of nursing to communication practice.

Nursing theory and conceptual model use to guide nurse–patient communication practices

Partnership in the nurse–patient relationship with recognition of patient autonomy is a recurring theme throughout popular nursing theory (Pearson *et al.*, 2000). This particular aspect of nursing has relevance for moving away from the medical, traditional and routine models of care (Pearson *et al.*, 2000). We selected theories for consideration in this chapter due to their popularity of use and their relevance to the topic under consideration. These are the Roper-Logan Tierney (RLT) conceptual model (Roper *et al.*, 1980, 1985, 1990, 1996, 2001), Orem's Self-Care Deficit Theory of Nursing (SCDNT) and Peplau's Conceptual Frame of Reference for Psychodynamic Nursing (Peplau, 1952, 1991).

The Roper-Logan-Tierney (RLT) model of nursing (Roper *et al.*, 1980, 1985, 1990, 1996, 2001) is both a conceptual model and a theory of nursing. It was developed in Edinburgh and is widely used throughout the UK and Ireland. Orem's Self-Care Deficit Nursing Theory (SCDNT) (Orem, 2001), is one of the most widely used theories in practice (Berbiglia, 2002). Although primarily a theory of nursing, Fawcett (1995) noted that the concepts and propositions of this theory can also be used at a practical (conceptual model) level;

and may be used, therefore, as a framework to guide specific nursing actions. Peplau's Conceptual Frame of Reference for Psychodynamic Nursing (Peplau, 1952, 1991) is a theory of nursing.

It is beyond the scope of the chapter to describe these models in their totality and reference to seminal texts is advised. The Roper-Logan-Tierney (RLT) model of nursing was described in original texts (Roper *et al.*, 1980, 1985, 1990, 1996, 2001) and other useful texts on the topic (Pearson *et al.*, 2000, Holland *et al.*, 2004). It is underpinned by a 'model of living' described by Roper *et al.* (2001, p. 13) who identified five main components of human living that constituted the 'main features of this highly complex phenomenon'. These concepts are interrelated and presented on Figure 2.2.

Roper *et al.* (2001) proposed that living involved the completion of 12 activities of living (ALs) (Figure 2.3). These ALs were the central focus of the model. It was the interaction and relationship between the ALs and the other components (Figure 2.4) that facilitated the notion of individuality as a discrete component to emerge (Roper *et al.*, 2001).

The nursing process (assess, plan, implement and evaluate) is used in conjunction with the RLT (Roper *et al.*, 2001). Persons requiring nursing care undergo an assessment in each of the ALs, with consideration for the factors influencing these activities, the dependence–independence continuum and lifespan

---

- Activities of Living (ALs)
- Lifespan
- Dependence/independence continuum
- Factors influencing the ALs
- Individuality in Living

Source: Adapted from Roper, N., Logan, W.W. and Tierney, A.J. (2001) *The Roper Logan Tierney Model of Nursing Based on Activities of Living*, London: Churchill Livingstone with permission from Elsevier.

Figure 2.2   The five main components of the Roper–Logan–Tierney (RLT) (2001) model of nursing

1. Maintaining a safe environment
2. Communicating
3. Breathing
4. Eating and drinking
5. Eliminating
6. Personal cleansing and dressing
7. Controlling body temperature
8. Working and playing
9. Mobilizing
10. Sleeping
11. Expressing sexuality
12. Dying

Source: Roper, N., Logan, W.W. and Tierney, A.J. (2001) *The Roper Logan Tierney Model of Nursing Based on Activities of Living*, London: Churchill Livingstone with permission from Elsevier.

Figure 2.3 The 12 Activities of Living used in the Roper–Logan–Tierney (RLT) (2001) model of nursing

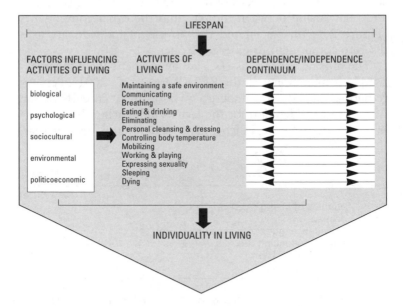

Source: Roper, N., Logan, W.W. and Tierney, A.J. (2001) *The Roper Logan Tierney Model of Nursing Based on Activities of Living*, London: Churchill Livingstone with permission from Elsevier.

Figure 2.4 The Model of Living

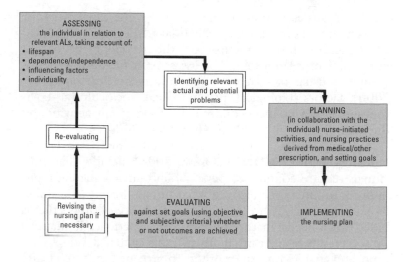

Source: Roper, N., Logan, W.W. and Tierney, A.J. (2001) *The Roper Logan Tierney Model of Nursing Based on Activities of Living*, London: Churchill Livingstone with permission from Elsevier.

Figure 2.5   Individualizing nursing as a dynamic process using the Roper–Logan–Tierney Model of Nursing

issues. Problems (actual or potential) are identified and transferred to a care plan, so that necessary nursing care may be planned, implemented and documented. At later stages of the nursing process the care given is evaluated. This process, which they describe as dynamic and continuous, is displayed in Figure 2.5.

Roper *et al.* (2001) emphasized the individual nature of this process of nursing and the necessity for patient participation, all elements of what we may begin to consider as patient-centred care. Their model also allows for specific assessment of individual needs and problems in the activity (AL) of communication, thus may be said to facilitate patient-centred communication. In their commentary on communication as an AL, Roper *et al.* (2001, p. 22) highlighted that this is 'a highly individual activity', however 'it is not the individual who is crucial, but the interpersonal relationship'. Thus introducing another important element in communication, the nurse–patient relationship.

Although description of the nature of the assessment for this activity emphasizes the individual nature of communication, there is little direction on the development of the nurse–patient relationship. The assessment focuses on identifying the usual pattern of communication (Pearson *et al.*, 2000), factors (biological, psychological, sociocultural, environmental and politicoeconomic) affecting this activity and the identification of problems (Iggulden, 2004).

The underlying assumptions of Orem's Self-Care Deficit Nursing Theory (SCDNT) (Orem, 2001) include: that individuals require continuous personal and environmental input in order to function effectively; that human *agency* (the ability to act deliberately), involves self-care and care of others that is based upon needs; mature humans can experience limitations on this (self-care and care of others); this agency develops over time, and enables oneself or others to provide inputs to ensure effective functioning.

The SCDNT incorporates three intertwining theories (Orem, 2001): self-care, self-care deficit and the theory of nursing systems. Self-care, Orem (2001) suggested, must be learned and performed deliberately. This theory assumes everyone develops and uses skills throughout their life to enable them to be able to take care of themselves and their dependents. The theory of self-care deficit explains that when people's needs for care exceed their own ability to meet these needs, people may require nursing care.

The *theory of nursing systems* brings together all the essential components of the SCDNT. It explains that nursing is a human action; formed by nurses through the exercise of their nursing agency for persons with health-derived or health-associated limitations in self-care or dependent care.

Therapeutic self-care is an essential element in the SCDNT. The nurse may assesses therapeutic self-care demand by analysing therapeutic self-care requisites in three distinct domains: universal, health deviation and developmental.

Universal self-care requisites are universally required goals that are met through self-care or dependent care. Eight self-care requisites common to all were identified by Orem (2001) and are displayed in Figure 2.6. Meeting the universal self-care requisites through self-care or dependent-care is

1. The maintenance of a sufficient intake of air
2. The maintenance of a sufficient intake of water
3. The maintenance of a sufficient intake of food
4. The provision of care associated with elimination processes
    and excrements
5. The maintenance of balance between activity and rest
6. The maintenance of balance between solitude and social
    interaction
7. The prevention of hazards to human life, human functioning,
    and human well being
8. The promotion of human functioning and development
    within social groups in accordance with human potential,
    known human limitations and the human desire to be normal

Source: Adapted from: Orem, D.E. (2001) *Nursing Concepts of Practice* (6th edn.) London, Mosby.

Figure 2.6   Universal Self-Care Requisites (Orem 2001)
Source: adapted from Peplau, H.E. (1991) *Interpersonal Relations in Nursing A Conceptual Frame of Reference for Psychodynamic Nursing*, New York: Springer.

an integral component of the daily living of individuals and groups.

A later addition to the model, *Developmental self-care requisites* are concerned with all aspects of human development. Orem (2001) outlined three sets of developmental requisites, the provision of conditions that promote development, engagement in self-development and interferences with development.

Health deviation self-care requisites are self-care requisites that exist for persons who are ill or injured, who have specific forms of pathological conditions or disorders, and who are undergoing medical diagnosis treatment.

The first stage for nurses when using this model is *assessment*. This 'calculation and design' of the therapeutic self-care demand requires an 'investigative process' Orem (2001, p. 247). Although not explicitly stated in the model, the nursing process underpins the operation of the model in practice. This information is transferred to a care plan.

Planning outlines the amount of care that an individual requires. It involves outlining the actions (related to human functioning and development) that the individual should perform or have performed by another within a specific time-frame.

Intervention, involves nursing systems, a series of deliberate (collaborative with patient) practical actions to meet patients' therapeutic self-care demands and to protect and promote patients' self-care agency (ability to meet their own needs) (Orem, 2001).

Within this nursing system, nursing care can be described and implemented on a continuum ranging from *wholly compensatory* (doing for the patient), *partly compensatory* (helping the patient to do for himself or herself) or *supportive-educative* (helping the patient learn to do for himself or herself).

Partnership is an explicit aspect of the use of SCDNT as a conceptual model in practice. Empowerment is also crucial. Rather than nursing care being regarded solely as providing direct care to another, Orem (2001) also highlighted the important nursing actions of supporting and educating patients. The development of the nurse–patient relationship was identified as crucial to this process (Orem, 2001). It is also essential for the full and participative involvement of patients in care as suggested.

 Exercise

Consider how conceptual models of nursing can improve your communication practices.

The development of a nurse–patient relationship was a fundamental component of Peplau's (1952, 1991) work. This Conceptual Frame of Reference for Psychodynamic Nursing held that the emphasis in nursing care was the growth of the patient through partnership with the nurse. This partnership (the nurse–patient relationship) evolves through distinct phases (Figure 2.7). During the *orientation* phase patients' individual educational needs are considered and addressed. Peplau (1991) specified nursing actions during this phase to

	Orientation	Identification	Exploitation	Resolution
Admission	••			
Intervention	••	••	••	
Recovery	••	••	••	••
Discharge			••	••

Figure   2.7 Overlapping   Phases   in   Nurse–Patient Relationships (Peplau 1991)

include acting as a resource person, as a listener and as a technical expert. The patient begins to identify their needs from the experience.

Exercise

Consider how you may identify patients' needs during the orientation phase.

In the next phase, *identification*, the patient may strongly identify with a nurse as the basis for the formation of the nurse–patient relationship. Peplau (1991, p. 37) outlined how both the patient and nurse 'make use' of this identification. Both the nurse and patient allow this developing professional relationship to form the basis of recovery. Once this identification takes place, Peplau (1991) suggested that a patient proceeds to a phase (*exploitation*) whereby he 'makes full use of the services offered to him'. The patient feels confident and able to utilize the resources available in the health care context. When goals have been achieved, *resolution* occurs and new goals are formed for discharge. Peplau (1991, p. 40) suggested that this phase will only occur through 'psychological mothering' and she described one aspect of the nurse role as 'surrogate'. While this language and thinking does appear outdated, the fundamental message is not: that a 'sustaining relationship' (1991, p. 40) is required between nurses and patients that allows identification of individual patient needs, action to address these needs and emotional support. Other roles identified by Peplau (1991) were: counsellor, resource, teacher, technical expert and leader.

Exercise

Consider how you may increase the likelihood of patient identification with the nurse during this phase.

The importance of the nurse–patient relationship within nursing was of crucial importance to Peplau (1991). Pearson *et al.* (2000, p. 170) noted that 'Peplau concentrates on developing the ideas of nursing and interpersonal processes she gives only cursory consideration to health and the environment'. The interpersonal relationship advocated by Peplau (1991) fosters patient recovery and rehabilitation but also allows the 'individuals to understand their health problems and to learn from their experience' (Pearson *et al.*, 2000 p. 170).

These notions are of particular relevance in today's health care setting. In a consumer driven era there is increasing emphasis on patient satisfaction with services. Although in many cases the procedural aspects of hospitalized care may have been intact, the literature abounds with research indicating that communication within the heath care setting is less than optimal. In addition, with the increasing use and publication of qualitative studies, there are many examples of the emotional consequences of hospitalization. Furthermore, there is increasing evidence that patients' educational needs are not always met in the hospital setting.

This model emphasizes and draws out the development of the nurse–patient relationship, which should become, as it was for Peplau (1991) the main focus of care. 'To Peplau, the essence of nursing is in thse interpersonal relationship between the nurses and the client' (Pearson *et al.*, 2000, p. 171). This one-to-one approach this may help to improve communication, information giving and emotional support given by nurses. Although there is a concern that over-involvement at a personal level may occur, there is an emphasis on professional closeness (Pearson *et al.*, 2000).

Peplau's (1991) theory of nursing is carried out through observation, communication and recording. The process is shown in Figure 2.8. The development of the interpersonal relationship between patient and nurse, aimed at developing

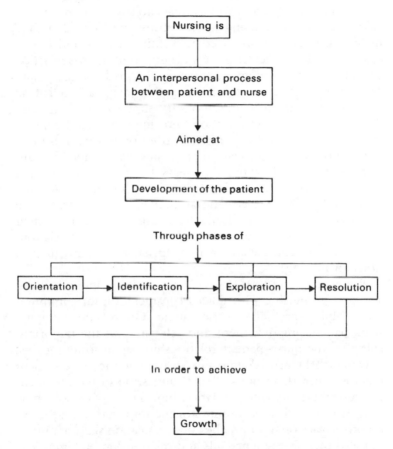

Source: Pearson, A., Vaughan, B. and Fitzgerald, M. (2000) *Nursing Models for Practice*, 2nd edn. London: Butterworth Heinemann, with permission from Elsevier.

Figure 2.8 A Diagramatic Representation of Peplau's Developmental Model

the patient, through the various phases identified, is a predominant theme in this book. The notion of therapeutic communication is continued and developed in the next chapter.

Although it is not readily acknowledged, nursing has freed itself only minimally, in some areas, from the medical model of care. Consideration of patients in terms of conditions and treatments limits the personal approach to care. It also fails to consider the greater social, emotional and psychological influences on health. There is also evidence to suggest that in some cases the focus of nursing is on getting the work done and nursing care is often reduced to routine, rituals and is task orientated. The effect of these working conditions is isolation of the patient. Although, ultimately the goals of the health care settings may be achieved, the patient may have deficits in terms of informational and emotional support.

Through a brief exploration of nursing theory and conceptual models and their potential contribution to care, it is obvious that this conceptualization of nursing represents a forward step in the holistic care of patients by nurses. As by their nature they consider the individual, health, nursing and the environment, they have made an immeasurable contribution towards the individualization of nursing. Furthermore, their focus on communication skills and the nurse–patient relationship as a core component of nursing has important implications for nursing.

Roper *et al.* (2001) suggested a very individualized approach to nursing with special consideration for communication ability/problems of the patient. Orem (2001) emphasized patient empowerment and self-care and the important role that the nurse–patient relationship has in fostering this. Peplau (1991) focused almost exclusively on the nurse–patient relationship with an unparalleled suggestion of the therapeutic contribution of this relationship. Description of these models in this chapter illuminates the importance that nurse theorists place on not only the communication skills of nurses, but also their assessment skills and relationship building. The use of each of these approaches to care will influence care management in different ways. However, fundamental to these approaches is the developing notion of therapeutic communication and patient-centred communication. It is only through the adoption of these principles that current gaps in service provision can be addressed and health care provision can become truly customer orientated and based on community and individual needs.

Key points

▶ Barriers to the development of patient-centred therapeutic communication include: failure to individualize nursing care; ritualistic nursing actions and lack of communication skills.

▶ Nursing theory can be used as a framework to conceptualize, describe and inform the unique contribution of nursing to health care provision.

▶ Nursing theory guides and informs nursing practice, thereby preventing ritualistic nursing.

▶ The integral role of communication and patient-centredness is a recurring theme in contemporary nursing theory that provides a nursing rather than medical model of care.

---

3 Therapeutic communication

Introduction

This chapter explores the concepts of therapeutic communication and patient-centred communication in nursing practice using psychological theories as a framework to develop the discussion. These theories are commonly used in nursing to provide explanations about human behaviour and when applied to the nurse–patient relationship, can help nurses use communication that is patient-centred, therapeutic and effective. Knowledge of these theories can also help nurses, as individuals and professionals, understand their own behaviour in the nurse–patient relationship by helping them become aware of themselves, their personal needs and personal reactions (O'Kelly, 1998, Gallop and O'Brien, 2003).

Sigmund Freud

The first of these theories relates to the work of Sigmund Freud who developed a model of personality that identified the *id*, the *ego* and the *superego* as the three main components of personality. The *id*, which is present at birth, is based on the pleasure principle. It represents the basic human need to satisfy certain desires, such as food, comfort and sleep, in order to survive. The *ego* develops as the infant grows in response to its environment and is based on the reality principle. In other words it balances the drive of the id in the context of reality, what is socially acceptable behaviour and in maintaining self-esteem. The *superego* is the third and perhaps most complex aspect to the development of personality that begins to develop as the child becomes an adolescent. It is concerned with the development of conscience and the incorporation of an individuals and society's sense of morality and forms the basis of values and beliefs that play an integral role in behaviour. Freud believed essentially that unconscious forces and desires drive human behaviour and these need to become conscious so that healthy relationships can occur (Dworetzky, 1997). While this detail may seem unrelated to explaining nurse–patient relationships, it does provide knowledge about human behaviour, the development of self through interaction with others and personal development (Gallop and O'Brien, 2003). This in turn encourages and enables nurses to develop an awareness of the various forces that influence nurse–patient relationships and in particular how their personal behaviour contributes to the relationship and whether or not it is a therapeutic relationship for the patient.

Freud believed that human behaviour and decision-making is unconsciously influenced by each individual's past experiences, feelings, values and beliefs. Freud introduced the concepts of transference and counter-transference as a means of explaining the underlying dynamic in an interaction. Transference, which is also sometimes referred to as projection, is described as behaviour in which individuals uncon sciously project seemingly inappropriate or irrational feelings/attitudes towards others that are based on previous personal experiences or relationships. In the context of the nurse–patient relationship this means for example that a patient communicates with a nurse based on a past relationship or experience that is unrelated to the present situation. Talking to a nurse may arouse feelings of anger in a patient who has unresolved issues in relation to the death of a parent. Counter-transference is the nurse's counter-reaction to the patient's transference and perhaps includes the nurse's own transference issues. Transference and counter-transference is clearly a two-way process in which a person transfers or projects their own thoughts, feelings, emotions and needs onto another person either consciously or unconsciously. This can result in a positive or negative interaction but ultimately, and depending on the nature of the transference or counter transference behaviours, it can influence the development of a therapeutic nurse–patient relationship (Gallop and O'Brien, 2003; O'Kelly, 1998). O'Kelly (1998) describes over-involvement and withdrawal as expressions of counter-transference in the nurse's behaviour. The relationship a nurse has with a patient may mirror positive or negative aspects of the relationship they had with their mother or father. However, recognition of responses as counter-transference represents a challenge for nurses as does the understanding of the possible impact of these responses on the development of the nurse–patient relationship. Once a patient is labelled as 'difficult' it means that from the nurses' perspective, they become the reason why the nurse–patient relationship is a negative one. This of course is not the case but it is only by examining their own behaviour and developing an awareness of transference and counter-transference responses that they use, that nurses can begin to have a clearer picture of how they can ensure that the relationships that they have with patients, regardless of their duration, can be therapeutic.

 Exercise

Think about one aspect of your parents' personality that evokes either positive or negative feelings in you. How does this part of their personality make you feel?

Next, think about a friend or partner and whether or not there is a link between a particular aspect of their personality that you react most strongly to and the one you identified in your parents. You may see a link immediately but if not, think about whether or not you have the same response and reaction to other people who exhibit the same aspect of personality that your parents did.

This type of exercise may help you to develop awareness about your personal behaviour and realize that often the way we respond to others is often more about ourselves than those with whom we are communicating.

Maslow

In contrast to Freud, psychologists from the humanistic school of thought, such as Maslow (1954) and Rogers

(1961), were of the view that people are driven by positive forces to achieve their full potential in life. People are thought to be basically good and trustworthy and prefer growth and love to aggression and destruction. In order to understand human behaviour, individuals need to be considered as a whole rather than trying to understand humans as a combination of parts. Maslow (1954) believed that humans have specific needs that drive them towards ultimately meeting and satisfying these needs. These needs are described as a hierarchy with physiological needs (food, water, sleep) being the most basic and one that is present at birth. As the infant grows to childhood; and then to adulthood, their needs develop to include: safety, the need to belong, the need for a positive self-esteem and finally the need for self-actualization. In order to reach this a person would need to have achieved fulfilment in the other stages.

According to Maslow (1954) very few people achieve self-actualization, which he describes as a 'journey' or way of life rather than a goal in life. In his research Maslow was concerned with identifying things that make humans different from each other. In terms of nursing practice, this theory is useful for explaining or determining when a patient is ready for a nursing intervention. For example if a nurse needs to change a dressing on a wound, they will ensure that the patient feels comfortable, warm, secure and pain-free prior to starting the dressing. Throughout the procedure the nurse talks to the patient about the progress of wound healing and answers any queries the patient may have. Following the procedure the nurse will discuss when the next dressing needs to be done and what activities the patient can do in the meantime to promote wound healing. The nurse will leave the patient feeling comfortable and secure.

Carl Rogers

Rogers' (1961) personality theory focuses on self-perception and self-concept as key aspects to understanding a person's personality and these emerge from interacting with others and feedback from others. He proposed that unlike Freud's theory, human behaviour is purposeful; individuals are free to make choices and develop their own personalities rather than being driven by unconscious forces or learned behaviour. Rogers (1969) also adapts the humanistic approach and introduces the 'person-centred' theory. This theory is concerned with understanding interpersonal interaction and Rogers (1969) identifies three key components of the person-centred theory. These are warmth, empathy and genuineness. Warmth is necessary for a relationship to develop and it refers to making an individual 'special' or showing that you respect them as an individual. To do this successfully, a person would need to exhibit unconditional positive regard towards others. This means having an innate respect for people that is non-judgemental. Empathy, which is regarded as a helping skill, will be discussed in detail in Chapter 4.

Genuineness is a concept that is difficult to describe. It is a perception that a person has about another because they perceive that person to communicate in an open, honest and sensitive manner. These qualities are imparted through the use of congruent behaviour, that is, the verbal language that a person uses matches their non-verbal language; and is the foundation stone of a therapeutic nurse–patient relationship. Some nurses find it easy to use these skills others may not. It can be a challenge to disregard our own views and feelings when caring for patients and accept them as unique individuals regardless of their background or illness. When a nurse labels a patient or passes judgement on them, they will be unable to communicate in a therapeutic or patient-centred way because they are focusing on their own views and feelings rather than the needs of the patient as a unique individual.

Martin Buber

Martin Buber (1958) presents the view that our reality is defined by the way we speak to each other. He suggests that people use two ways of communicating: I–It and I–Thou. The I–It relationship occurs when we view people and issues objectively. An example of this in nursing is when a patient is described as 'the fractured hip in bed four'. Instead of sharing themselves with patients, understanding them and talking to them as individuals, nurses consider it important to keep a 'distance' between themselves and the patients that they care for. It is a relationship that demonstrates separateness and detachment. In contrast, the I–Thou relationship is one of mutuality and reciprocity. In the nurse–patient relationship this means that the nurse and the patient respect each other as individuals with equal commitment and responsibility in the relationship. The individualized approach to nursing care as advocated by nurse theorists is in keeping with this theory. However, according to Buber (1958), each person needs to enter the I–Thou relationship without preconditions. This can be a challenge for nurses because of how they are socialized. Traditionally nurses were not supported or encouraged by health care organizations to establish therapeutic relationships with patients. One possible reason for this is to reduce staff stress levels by encouraging nurses to distance themselves from difficult emotional situations (Menzies, 1970). It seems that although nurses are no longer encouraged to distance themselves from patients, this practice remains in nursing culture. Also just as nurses are socialized, patients too are socialized and have preconceived stereotyped ideas of the role of the nurse. Patients, depending on their past experiences of being a patient, level of education, knowledge or personal views on health and illness, may wish to be active participants in planning and organizing their care. On the other hand some patients may take on a passive role and rely on the nurses and other health care professionals to make decisions regarding their care. However, an awareness by nurses of their own and possibly patients' preconceived ideas, may compensate for this and by entering into the relationship with the I–Thou attitude or even Rogers patient-centred view then nurses may be able to use their communication skills to establish what level of control a patient wishes to have over every aspect of their care. For example, a patient may retain the role of meeting their own hygiene needs and actively discuss their illness and plan of care with the nurse, but yet may resist giving their own insulin injection. It requires sensitivity and empathy on the part of the nurse to recognize when a patient is not comfortable participating in their own care and provide an opportunity for the patient to verbalize their concerns and fears about participating. By providing opportunities where patients feel comfortable about voicing their concerns and do not feel a nuisance or that they are holding up the busy nurse, nurses will be able to provide more effective nursing care where the advice and education that they give to patients is individualized and meets the specific needs of the patient.

Patient-centred communication

Patient-centred care is a concept that nurses are familiar with because it is often referred to in nurse education and nursing theory as the context in which nurses should plan, organize and provide patient care. Patient-centred communication is defined as 'communication that invites and encourages the patient to participate and negotiate in decision-making regarding their own care' (Langwitz *et al.*, 1998, p. 230). While participation and negotiation are regarded as key elements in patient-centred communication, it could be argued that the term implies that the balance of power and control in this relationship lies with the nurse. However, for communication to be patient-centred, power and control need to be shared equally between the nurse and the patient. This can be a challenge for nurses because, as mentioned in relation to Buber's I–Thou theory, nurses are socialized by the culture and organization of nurse education and health care management into a task-centred approach to patient care. This means that nurses adopt a communication style that focuses on the completion of tasks relating to patients rather than communicating with the patient as a person with their own individual needs.

Rogers (1961) views certain qualities in a nurse, such as warmth, genuineness and empathy as a prerequisite for communication to be patient-centred. This implies that it is not enough to invite or encourage a patient to participate and negotiate in planning their own care, as this will only be successful if it is done within the context of warmth, genuineness and empathy. Buber's I–Thou theory that mutual respect as individuals, equal commitment and responsibility are essential ingredients in a relationship is communicated in the nurse–patient relationship through warmth, genuineness and empathy. The nurse will know by the feedback from the patient whether or not they perceive the nurse to have a genuine concern for them as an individual. They will respond by smiling and telling the nurse about themselves. Nursing has moved away from the delivery of nursing care through task allocation, for example, one nurse doing the 'obs' and another doing dressings, to one of patient allocation, team nursing or primary care. These systems of care although based on a holistic and patient-centred school of thought, do not result in patients receiving patient-centred care.

A key point in the successful development of a patient-centred relationship is the value that nurses place on this relationship. A nurse, although working within a patient-centred system of patient care such as team nursing, may have the I–It view of patients and view the planning and organization of patient care as a series of tasks to be completed within the duration of a working day. These tasks may be completed efficiently and competently, however this approach can leave the patient feeling very detached and even lonely. A narrative from a study by McCabe (2004) on nurse–patient communication from a patient's perspective demonstrates this: 'the only time they'd sit down was when they were taking your blood pressure . . . they'd sit there for a few minutes and then move on to the next patient'. When asked if the nurses spoke to him when they sat down, this participant said 'very little, I think that's the slackest part but as I said, they can't be sitting down talking with patients – I'd say they'd be neglecting their own work then.' This patient does not regard himself as being connected with the work of the nurse, the relationship appears very detached and the patient very isolated. The nurse on the other hand feels satisfied or relieved that she is getting through her workload and appears to be competent and efficient. In relation to Freud's view on counter-transference, it is only by bringing our communication behaviours into our awareness that we can begin to use responses that are patient-centred rather than responses based on personal feelings and experiences and needs.

Maslow's (1954) hierarchy of needs advocates the recognition of the person as a 'whole' with specific needs, starting with physiological needs (food, water, sleep, warmth) as the foundations for achieving other needs, such as, safety, the need to belong, the need for a positive self-esteem and finally the need for self-actualization. This provides a framework for nurses in prioritizing the needs of a patient. However, often in nursing we talk about the physical and psychological needs of patients as almost separate parts of the person but as the following narrative from McCabe's (2004) study demonstrates, they are inextricably linked: 'I didn't have a shower for the first two days, it just would have taken somebody sensitive enough to understand . . . I mean you can imagine what you feel like when you can't even wash yourself.' The lack of attention to the physical needs of this patient left her feeling frustrated and unable to trust the nurses. By attending to and anticipating the physical needs of a patient, nurses are also attending to their psychological needs but for this to be patient-centred requires that the patient perceives the nurse to be warm, genuine and empathetic. If this does not happen then the patient will not trust the nurse and may appear withdrawn or unfriendly from the nurses' perspective whereas they may just be lonely and feeling isolated. When a patient feels this way, it is very difficult for the nurse to establish a positive relationship. As 'The Comforting Interaction-Relationship Model' (Morse *et al.*, 1997) suggests, the duration of a relationship is not a factor in whether it is patient-centred or not. It is to do with whether the nurse views the patient in a holistic way as an unique individual and can communicate in a warm, genuine and empathetic manner in meeting the needs of the patient. This is done through our verbal and non-verbal communication and will be explored in detail in the following chapters.

Developing awareness of and changing communication behaviour

The process of becoming aware of how we communicate as individuals is a challenging one. It requires that nurses discuss the interactions between themselves and their patients with other nursing colleagues or it may be more comfortable initially to discuss issues with someone unrelated to work. You might find it easier to do this on a one-to-one basis at first but as you become better at talking about how you communicate and contributed (good and bad) to interactions with patients, it may be more beneficial to do this with a group of work colleagues that you trust and regard as role models. The focus of these discussions should be to determine whether the interaction was patient-centred or not. If as a group it is agreed that this was not patient-centred it is essential to determine why it was not and what factors prevented this from happening. Before ending the discussion it is imperative for the development of patient-centred communication that the group decide what specific communication behaviours would have facilitated patient-centred communication in this interaction and it is these interactions that the nurse needs to remember and use consciously in future interactions with patients.

Therapeutic communication

Knowledge of how human beings behave and what motivates human behaviour is important for providing nurses and other health care professionals with an understanding of why therapeutic communication is important when caring for people and will also help in using therapeutic skills more effectively (Wondrak, 1998). The term 'therapeutic' is defined as 'relating to the healing arts or to the curing of disease contributing towards or performed to improve health or general well-being' (*Chambers Dictionary*, 2003) or as 'causing someone to feel happier and more relaxed or to be more healthy (*Cambridge Advanced Learner's Dictionary*). It is a term associated primarily with counselling or psychotherapy that perceives communication as the primary channel for being therapeutic. The communication skills required to have a therapeutic effect are the same as those that are sometimes used between family members, friends and colleagues in everyday situations. The difference between ordinary everyday communication and therapeutic communication between a nurse and a patient lies in the professional context and motivation of the nurse towards providing high quality nursing care for people with individual needs.

Therapeutic communication is a term that is used widely in nursing and in relation to counselling and psychotherapy. In order to provide clarity, the meaning of the term in both contexts will be explored. In counselling and psychotherapy the concept of therapeutic communication requires the presence of a person (counsellor or psychotherapist) who is perceived as having specialist knowledge, experience and communication skills. The sole purpose of therapeutic communication in this context is to encourage and facilitate the development of communication skills in those with immature or disturbed behaviour to form stable and satisfying social relations (Ruesch, 1973). This takes place in the context of a professional relationship in which the counsellor or therapist provides specific time, attention and venue for the client or patient.

Since Peplau's (1952) work, nurse theorists and nurse educators have referred to the importance of nurses developing a therapeutic relationship with patients. The aim of nurses using therapeutic communication skills is not to treat or cure a disease or disorder. It is to provide a sense of well-being for patients by making them feel relaxed and secure. This helps to establish rapport and trust between the nurse and the patient. These are essential ingredients for the development of a positive nurse–patient relationship. Therapeutic communication results in a focused and purposeful relationship established by the nurse in order to assess, plan, implement and evaluate the care needed by a patient. This benefits the patient and the nurse through the achievement of mutually agreed outcomes of care that are based on the patient's individual physical and psychological needs. The duration of the relationship is not a factor in establishing a therapeutic nurse–patient relationship. What is required is that the nurse is competent in the nursing skills required to deliver care safely. Patients observe nurses not only to determine if they are nice people and trustworthy but also to see if they are competent at nursing skills, using equipment and anticipating their needs. Patients need to be able to trust nurses to be aware of specific care that they need and also need to know that nurses can deliver this care using the necessary equipment and skills competently and safely. This is another example of how the physical care of a patient impacts on their psychological well-being. If they do not feel that the nurse is a safe practitioner they will not trust them and this will impact negatively on the development of the nurse–patient relationship regardless of the communication approach used by the nurse.

If therapeutic communication is about making a patient feel relaxed and secure then another essential ingredient in establishing a therapeutic relationship is patient-centred communication. As discussed earlier this makes patients feel that they are respected as individuals, that nurses have a genuine concern for their well-being and that they have control over the care they receive. The absence of a patient-centred approach to communication will inhibit the development of a therapeutic nurse–patient relationship. The key characteristics of therapeutic nurse–patient communication include a perception of caring, openness, warmth, genuineness, empathy and purpose on the part of the nurse. For undergraduate nursing students and newly qualified nurses, therapeutic communication may be perceived as a complex and time consuming process. Within the modern health care structure, the time a patient spends in hospital is often very short, for example, in day surgery facilities or five-day admission units. Although patients' needs may vary between being complex or emotionally difficult to deal with or very straightforward, the majority want the best treatment possible, delivered in a context that is helpful, positive and meets their specific needs. Even in emergency departments where nurse–patient relationships are of very short duration and often very intense, the most effective therapeutic communication skills are smiling, some eye contact, a calm steady tone of voice and open, honest communication. However, what is required is that nurses are aware of their own communication abilities and limitations and when patients need specialized therapeutic communication, nurses will discuss this with the patient and their doctor. As discussed previously the communication skills required to be therapeutic are no different to those used by people in ordinary everyday situations. These include verbal and non-verbal communication skills such as, listening, questioning, observation, and touch and will be discussed in detail in the next chapter.

Key points

▶ Psychological theories are useful in explaining the concept of patient-centredness.

▶ Theories by psychologists such as, Maslow (1954), Rogers (1961) and Freud can help nurses understand and become aware of their own behaviour and that of others.

▶ The development of a positive patient-centred relationship depends largely on the values held by nurses in relation to their role as nurses in the provision of holistic and individualized care.

▶ Therapeutic communication is focused and purposeful and makes patients feel relaxed and secure.

▶ Nurses need to be caring, open, warm, genuine, empathic and purposeful in order to communicate therapeutically.

PART II

The communication process
in nursing

4 Communication skills

Introduction

Communication skills are often classified as verbal and non-verbal with verbal, or the spoken word, being regarded as a key component in delivering a message. However, according to Argyle (1990) in an interaction, words make up 7 per cent of a message; tone, tempo and syntax make up 38 per cent; and body language makes up 35 per cent. This implies that although sometimes it is essential to use appropriate words when sending a message, how we send the message is a great deal more important than the words we use.

> **Exercise**
>
> When was the last time you were aware of giving someone a dirty look?
> Why did you give the dirty look?
> How did people respond to you?
> Did you get what you wanted?

This is an example of negative communication and highlights that just because we do not speak does not mean that we are not communicating.

Those skills that are generally described as basic communication skills include listening, questioning, body language and paralinguistics. However, it is probably more accurate to say that these communication skills and others that we will look at in this chapter are best defined as *core* communication skills rather than basic. *Core* communication skills are skills that most human beings have but individuals use these skills in various ways across many different contexts and with different levels of ability. The term *basic* denotes skills that are simple and easy to achieve and in a way this term is appropriate because most of us are born with the ability to listen, ask questions and use our bodies to communicate. This natural ease with which most humans develop communication skills from birth may explain why we perceive these skills as basic and even common sense. This perception can also be the reason why communication between people is sometimes very effective and positive, and other times it is ineffective, difficult and negative. Because it is perceived as a natural phenomenon, people generally do not think about how they communicate with others and feel that the way they communicate is beyond their control. Personality is often linked with the way a person communicates. It is perceived as a permanent aspect of our character, and therefore cannot be changed. Developing your communication skills is not about changing your personality; it is about developing and adapting your behaviour and responses in interactions in order to communicate positively and effectively with others.

In Chapter 1 you were asked to think about what communication is. You may have found this difficult because you do not generally think about communication and probably almost never discuss your communication skills with another person. We are generally much better at critically examining other people's communication skills that our own! However communication is a complex process that requires the use of core communication skills within many interactions throughout a day. The appropriate and effective use of these skills requires practice. This can be a challenge initially because we so rarely think consciously about how we communicate; therefore, practising these skills seems difficult and false. Developing effective communication skills is a similar process to acting. You learn your lines and you decide how your character should behave when delivering the lines. When learning to communicate, the purpose of this acting is not to be false or dishonest with others, it is to learn about and practise using specific communication skills appropriately and effectively in many different contexts. Like any skill (for example, playing a musical instrument) to do it well, you need to practise regularly and you get better every time you practise. Eventually you will be able to play a piece of music without thinking about it but you will not succeed unless you want to learn how to play the instrument. The same goes for learning to communicate well, you will not succeed unless you are prepared to examine your current communication behaviour and consciously learn and practice new communication skills and develop and focus the skills that you already have.

Exercise

Ask a person who knows you well (for example, a family member, partner or friend) to tell you what they think of your communication skills. You may have to tell them what you mean by communication because, like most people, they do not generally think about what communication is and may not know what information you are looking for. You might find it useful to ask them to rate your skills from 0–100 but they will need to explain their answers.

Most of us think we are better communicators than we are, so be prepared for the answer!

Communication is an integral part of nursing and, therefore, needs to be considered carefully and on a personal and professional basis by all nursing students. In order to use communication skills in a patient-centred way, nurses need not only to learn about and practise communication skills, they also need to have certain professional characteristics. These include genuineness, warmth and the ability to be empathetic. These characteristics come naturally to some people but others have to work at developing these characteristics by being non-judgemental towards patients, accepting patients as unique individuals and developing awareness of their own communication ability.

Establishing rapport

Communication skills such as listening, questioning, touch, paraphrasing and body language are used specifically by nurses in developing a trusting relationship or what is often referred to as *rapport* with patients. This is the foundation stone of a positive nurse–patient relationship and is worth spending time on when you meet a patient for the first time. First impressions count so it is important to introduce yourself, smile, lean towards the patient look directly at them and begin the interaction with an open ended question such as, 'how are you today?' (Williams, 2001). These communication behaviours convey warmth and genuineness to patients (Caris-Verhallen *et al.*, 1999). Appearances also matter. Patients observe the physical appearance of the nurse, for example how she wears her uniform and the expression on her face, and based on their own personal values and beliefs they will decide if a nurse looks like a *good* person and, therefore, trustworthy. This only takes a few seconds and influences the patient's initial response; therefore, the nurse needs to be aware of the message that her appearance is sending to patients. If a nurse looks untidy she may be perceived as disinterested, lazy and even incompetent even if this is not the case. Awareness of the non-verbal messages we send to others is essential, as it will often provide an explanation as to why people respond to us the way they do.

Listening

Listening is one of the most important of the non-verbal communication skills but its value is often underestimated. Hearing what another person is saying to us is just a small part of listening, remember, non-verbal communication makes up most of an interaction. Furthermore, we may hear what somebody is saying to us but that doesn't mean that we are actively listening. When you actively listen to another person it means that you are demonstrating your commitment to them as an unique individual, you want to help or comfort them, you want to understand them and you want to learn something or you may just want to enjoy their company (McKay *et al.*, 1995). Active listening requires that you give the other person your complete attention. This is conveyed primarily through the use of body language with minimal verbal interaction. 'You must be silent if you wish to listen to another, to listen with openness. This involves silencing not only your mouth but also your mind' (Perry, 1996, p. 9). Gibbons (1993) suggested that nurses find it difficult to be silent because their work is so action-oriented. This does not bode well for nurses' ability to actively listen to their patients. Silence is not an unresponsive communication. It is a skill, which, if used appropriately, gives patients a sense of time to think and talk. It also gives time to the nurse to respond in an appropriate and patient-centred way. The following steps may help you to develop your active listening skills:

- When the other person speaks to you, look at them with an open and interested expression on your face. This may be frustrating if you are busy and do not feel like it. It requires a conscious effort on your part to stop thinking about what you were doing and stop wondering when you will get back to it.
- Allow the person to speak without interrupting them and as they speak take note of how they are speaking and the body language they use. Awareness of this will provide you with more information about what they are feeling and what they are trying to say even though the words they use may not reflect this. Use some eye contact and prompts such as nodding your head to encourage them to speak freely and develop their thoughts.
- When you respond make sure that you reflect their feelings and that your facial expression and tone are appropriate and match what you are trying to say. You may need to clarify what they have said by asking questions and summarizing what they said. This does not send the message that you were not listening to them, instead it demonstrates that you are interested in ensuring that you understood the message correctly and you are trying to grasp fully what they said.
- Observe the feedback that you receive from the other person, if they seem happy with what you said or try to continue the conversation, then you can be sure that you have interpreted their words and body language correctly.

Feedback and clarification are two key characteristics of active listening. A third is paraphrasing (McKay *et al.*, 1995). Paraphrasing is repeating something that someone else said in your own words. In order to repeat what you have just heard you need to listen carefully. This demonstrates to others that you have been listening; therefore, you are interested in what they are saying. Paraphrasing prevents misunderstanding and misinterpretation of information and encourages communication that is open. In other words, you are so intent on listening to another person that you forget to be judgemental or you don't feel that you need to interrupt to say what you want to say.

 Exercise

Ask a friend or partner to tell you how their day went at work in detail. When they are finished repeat what they told you in your own words. Don't be too surprised at what you leave out or get confused! If you get it right and leave nothing out, think about whether you listened differently to the way you normally listen to patients – be honest with yourself!

Others perceive this type of communication behaviour as genuine behaviour. It is open, non-judgemental and your body language is congruent with the words that you use. In nursing, active listening is often regarded by nurses as a time-consuming process. This is not the case, and if a nurse is genuinely interested in a patient and what they have to say, active listening can be used effectively in even the briefest and most transient of encounters. However, instead of actively listening to patients, nurses can appear to be listening to patients in that they respond to what the patient says in a friendly and appropriate manner but they do not stop what they are doing or look directly at the patient when they respond. They may continue to adjust the intravenous line beside the patient or document the patient's vital signs or fluid intake without ever looking directly at them. This is false listening and gives the patient the message that the nurse is too busy to talk to them so they refrain from asking too many questions or discussing their care.

Scenario 1

A patient is lying in bed at 10am and would like to have a shower, however an intravenous infusion is in progress and there is still a small amount of fluid remaining to be infused. The alarm sounds on the infusion pump so the patient rings the nurse call bell to get a nurse's attention. A few minutes later a nurse enters the room and turns off the alarm. She says in a friendly voice 'I'll be back in a few minutes to deal with that for you' and leaves quickly. The patient waits for her return but after 20 minutes assumes that the nurse has forgotten because she is so busy. The alarms on the infusion pump sound again so the patient rings the nurse call bell once more. The same nurse returns and as responds to the alarm she says in a friendly and apologetic voice 'I am sorry about earlier on, I got caught up doing something and didn't get back to you, I'll just go and finish what I was doing and come straight back'. The patient says 'that's fine nurse and maybe you could help me to the shower then?' as the nurse leaves the room. 'Of course' the nurse says and is gone.

Scenario 2

A patient is lying in bed at 10am and would like to have a shower, however an intravenous infusion is in progress. The alarm sounds on the infusion pump so the patient rings the nurse call bell to get a nurse's attention. A few minutes later a nurse enters the room. She smiles at the patient and turns off the alarm. She looks at the patient and says, 'I'll be back in ten minutes to deal with that for you.' The patient says, 'that's great and maybe you could assist me with a shower then'. 'Yes certainly and perhaps after the shower you might like me to escort you on a walk down the corridor?' The patient nods her head and smiles in agreement and starts to gather things from her locker for the shower. The nurse returns ten minutes later as arranged.

The nurse in both of these scenarios was friendly and responded to the call bell quickly. However, in scenario 1, the patient was left feeling let down and possibly frustrated by the nurse because, although friendly, the nurse did not return when she said she would and she did not look directly at the patient throughout the interaction. This is an example of false listening and can be perceived by the patient as detachment or disinterest. The patient will find it difficult to trust this nurse and will probably stop the next nurse that comes into the room and ask her to help him have a shower. The nurse in the second scenario was friendly, but she also looked directly at the patient, smiled and in a very informal way, negotiated a short-term plan of care that met both their needs. This patient trusted the nurse because he knew he would obtain assistance with the shower and be able to take a walk when the nurse returned. This is an example of active listening that is patient-centred communication. As a student or junior staff nurse, you might have experienced similar feelings when trying to get the attention of a senior staff member. You ask a question once and if you don't get a response that you trust, you are less likely to approach that person again!

 Exercise

Have you ever been in a supermarket and gone through the checkout, paid for your groceries and said goodbye and thank you to the person at the checkout without looking directly at them? If you can't remember or don't know, next time you go in make a conscious effort to look at the person when you speak to them. If it feels odd, then you know that not looking directly at them is your normal behaviour. After this exercise think about how the person at the checkout responded when you looked directly at them and how this made you feel.

Exercise

Imagine being in a restaurant or a pub chatting to a friend. You have your back to the door and your friend is facing the door. You both have a good time chatting away but every now and then your friend looks over your shoulder towards the door. This is irritating and you start looking in the same direction and ask her what she's looking at. 'Nothing' she answers and continues talking. How does this make you feel?

Now think of a person that you do not normally pay much attention to or just pretend to listen to because you do not like them and find them boring. Next time you meet them try active listening and afterwards think about how it changed the pattern of the type of interactions you had previously with that person. You probably won't feel any different about the other person but will have had a much more positive experience

Touch

Physical touches can be a very powerful communication strategy when helping patients meet their physical needs and actively listening to another person.

- It can be empathetic by demonstrating understanding and support and can consequently alleviate patient anxiety and worry (Wondrak, 1998)
- Touch can also provide comfort and security for patients who are distressed or perhaps scared about their future.
- Touch can add meaning or emphasis to the spoken word.

Touch can be classified as *instrumental* touch or *expressive* touch (McCann and McKenna, 1993). Instrumental touch is the physical touch required to complete a task related to the physical needs of a patient. This is also referred to as functional touch.

Expressive touch is regarded as spontaneous and connecting with the patient as an individual on an emotional and possibly spiritual level (McCann and McKenna, 1993;

Routasalo, 1999). However, the findings from research on the use of physical touch in nursing vary widely. Routasalo (1999) suggests that this may be because the experience of touch for individuals is so subjective and contextually driven that it is extremely difficult to identify general experiences. In conjunction with other communication behaviours such as eye contact, smiling and speech, touch can have a calming and comforting effect on patients. However, not all touch will have this effect. The issue for nurses is how to know if a patient wants or is responding positively to touch. It is, therefore, important to observe the feedback from the patient. If they withdraw from a touch to the arm or shoulder then they are probably uncomfortable or may not trust the nurse. Respect for patients' personal and cultural difference will help prevent situations that are uncomfortable for both the nurse and the patient. Active listening is also a key element in accurately identifying if touch is appropriate or not.

Read the situation below for example:

> *Nurse*: Let me help you change those pyjamas
> *Patient*: Thanks, oooh, your hands are cold (with a laugh)
> *Nurse*: Yes, everyone tells me that, but you know what they say? Cold hands – Warm heart (laughing)

This exchange is open and friendly but the nurse has not listened to what the patient was saying. The nurse should have responded by apologizing and then running her hands under warm water to warm them up. Has anyone ever put a cold hand on you? You respond very quickly and move out of their reach! Well that's how a patient wants to react but can't because they need the nurse's help.

The way in which nurses use touch is influenced by their age, sex, culture, education level, and the part of the body to be touched, so even if you are not the type of person that generally uses expressive touch that does not mean that you do not communicate a message to patients when you touch them. Instrumental touch can also be calming and comforting for patients. This is because patients will feel the intention of your touch in the way that you deliver physical care. If your hands are warm and your touch is relaxed and smooth, with

eye contact and appropriate verbal cues, this will transmit a
positive feeling to patients. Any combination of jerky move-
ments along with cold hands and a 'busy' persona will transmit a more negative feeling to patients.

 Exercise

Try this with a friend or work colleague:
First shake hands and, as you do, take note of how their
skin feels against yours. Is it warm, hot, cold, cool, smooth,
rough, sweaty, firm grip or weak grip? Then ask the other
person to tell you how your hand felt to them.
The purpose of this exercise is to develop awareness of the
experience of touch for you and patients and how it can
influence responses in an interaction.

Questioning

Questioning is another core communication skill that we use
to meet many communication goals. These include:

- starting a conversation or keeping a conversation going;
- gaining information about others – this can be broad or
  specific;
- increasing our knowledge;
- encouraging participation and involvement in group
  discussions;
- encouraging others to reflect, evaluate and be critical;
- determining the level of knowledge in others; and
- control conversations.

The achievement of any of these goals requires the use of one
or more types of questions. They are classified as open, closed
and circular questions; and questions are classified according
to the amount of information required in response to the
question asked.

Open questions

Open questions are questions that give the respondent the opportunity to give as much or as little information as they wish when responding to a question. Asking open questions in an atmosphere that is relaxed and comfortable for patients encourages them to talk freely and for longer periods. Questions of this type help to build rapport between the nurse and patient. Open questions usually start with 'how', 'what' or 'please tell me about'.

Examples of open-ended questions include:

How are you feeling today?
What do you think of your new medication?
Please tell me about the history of your injury . . .

Open questions can also begin with 'why', for example:

Patient: I didn't go to the doctor until my son called to see me and insisted upon taking me.
Nurse: Why didn't you go to the doctor?

This seems like a reasonable question to ask and it is an important one, however the use of the word 'why' can make the patient feel that they did something wrong or that they need to justify their actions. Questions starting with 'why' can also be perceived as aggressive. Another way of asking the same question is:

Patient: I didn't go to the doctor until my son called to see me and insisted upon taking me.
Nurse: It sounds like you must have been very unwell?

In nursing, open questions can be used to determine a patient's cognitive ability, recall and their understanding of their care. If a patient is finding it difficult to respond to an open question, prompts, paraphrasing and repeating can be used to encourage the patient to continue talking. When open questions are used at the outset of an interaction, they can provide broad information and the nurse may need to use closed questions to clarify points and elicit specific information.

Closed questions

Closed questions need a limited and specific response. Examples of closed questions include:

Who is your next of kin?
What is your name?
Do you have a pain in your chest?

Closed questions can also be useful in the initial stages of the nurse–patient relationship to get someone talking or 'break the ice'. However, if used excessively, closed questions can limit the contribution of the patient to the interaction and result in the nurse controlling the scope and length of the conversation. This type of communication occurs frequently in nursing because nurses are busy and usually have a limited amount of time to spend with patients and closed questioning allows nurses to get specific information quickly. However, it does not encourage patients to talk, voice any concerns that they may have or contribute to the conversation generally. It is not patient-centred communication, instead it is task-centred, that is, it allows nurses to interact with patients at a very functional level and with the aim of getting the information they need so that they can proceed with completing any other work that they may have to do.

A combination of open and closed questions that is weighted towards open questions is the best option in nurse–patient communication. Following the patient's primary response to a question, the nurse can ask a probing or clarifying question. This allows nurses to get the specific information that they need and also encourages patients to talk while at the same time demonstrating the nurse's interest in listening to what patients have to say (Hargie and Dickson, 2004). The result is that patients feel valued and cared for as individuals. A rapport develops and this lays the foundation for a positive nurse–patient relationship.

When a nurse asks a patient a question, she needs to listen carefully to the answer the patient gives. The patient may avoid answering the question because the subject matter distresses them or because they did not understand the question. The patient may answer the question but the answer may seem vague or incongruent with the patient's behaviour. The following is an example of how questioning can go wrong:

> *Nurse*: Hi John, has that injection lessened your pain, it should be working by now?
> *Patient*: Eh, yes I think it is (patient appears restless and is finding it difficult to get comfortable)
> *Nurse*: Are you sure John, you don't seem to be comfortable?
> *Patient*: Well actually the injection hasn't made any difference; I'm still in a lot of pain!

The nurse in this scenario asked a very leading question. She implied that the injection should be working and that the patient should be feeling better. The patient, therefore, found it difficult to tell the nurse that the analgesia had not worked and probably felt that if they said nothing and waited a little longer, it would work. In this instance the nurse noticed the patient's incongruent behaviour and realized that he was still in pain. However, leading questions can result in incorrect or misleading responses. The other interesting aspect to this scenario is that even though the nurse asked a leading question, it is apparent that patients often try to give the answer that they think the nurse wants to hear. This is another reason why open questions are more patient-focused than closed questions.

Sometimes patients do not understand the question because of the terminology used. So simple language is essential, as are questions that are not lengthy or convoluted. Compare the following examples:

> Did you have your first surgery last year when you came in with the perforated ulcer or was that when you needed the laparotomy in 1999?

or

> Tell me everything about your illness from day one.

It is also very helpful for patients if nurses tell them why they are asking the questions and what they are going to do with the information. For example:

Hello my name is Jane and I'm going to be admitting you today. I need to ask you some questions that you may have been asked already but I will be recording this information in your nursing notes. This information will be used to identify your needs and help develop a plan of nursing care for you.

The type of question you use should be linked with the ability of the patient to answer. This will be determined by their level of understanding of their illness, level of education and how well or unwell they are. Closed questions are more effective for patients who are unwell or have lower intelligence (Hargie and Dickson, 2004). Open questions on the other hand result in responses that are more accurate, detailed and engaging for the person asking the questions.

Like any other aspect of communication it is important to think about what type of questions to use before beginning. This is influenced by the type of information you want, and why you want the information. You may just be asking the patient where they are from because you are interested in them and because you want to get to know them. You also need to choose the language of the question carefully and be very clear in the way that you speak when asking questions. The feedback or response from the patient will tell you whether your question was clear and understood. If you find that the patient does not understand you or misinterprets the question, the problem is more likely to do with how the question was asked than the person misunderstanding or misinterpreting the question.

Information giving

Patients are often reassured when they are given information about their illness, plan of care, and length of time they will be in hospital and how they can cope at home. However, patients can become stressed or even more anxious if they are given too much information over a short period of time. The type of information a patient needs depends on their level of intelligence, education, previous experience and knowledge of their illness. It can be difficult for a nurse to assess this quickly so a good rule of thumb is always ask the patient to repeat in their own words what you just told them or what they read in the information sheet. This should not be said in a patronizing way and should be preceded by an explanation as to why you are asking them to repeat it.

Written information should always be provided with verbal information where possible. This is because most patients experience some level of anxiety when in hospital or they may be distracted because most information is given to patients on the day of discharge or in the preceding days. They may receive information about the drugs they will need to take when discharged, outpatient appointments, how to look after their wound or dressing, what they should do and what they shouldn't do. It is hardly surprising that they forget what the nurse has said to them. Furthermore patients are often thinking about how they will cope at home or are busy getting their things together to pack, therefore, they miss important information. Preparing patients for discharge well in advance may help patients remember instructions. Giving information to patients when their next-of-kin or relative is present may also be helpful.

Paralinguistics

'It's not what you say, it's how you say it!'

Paralinguistics are non-verbal communication elements that refer to the tone and pitch of the voice and accent of the speaker and the speed at which they speak. Either on its own or in conjunction with the spoken word paralinguistics are used to express attitudes or emotions. They can also complement or contradict the spoken word. A simple statement can be interpreted in many different ways depending on the tone and pitch of the voice and also the emphasis of the speaker, for example the following statement made by a nurse to a patient: 'Wake up, it is time for your medication.' If this is said using a quiet, soft and low tone of voice, the patient will more than likely wake up and take their medication. However if this is said in a louder, more high-pitched voice, the experience will be quite different for the patient. As you can imagine if you were the patient, it is irritating and demonstrates a lack of consideration on the part of the nurse.

Accents play a key role in establishing a nurse–patient relationship. A query about the accent of the nurse is often a starting point or an icebreaker when a patient meets a nurse for the first time. If the patient or nurse is familiar with the accent it can help them to be more comfortable with each other and help the relationship to develop positively. However, it can also result in labelling and/or prejudice if the patient or nurse has preconceived ideas about the culture or class associated with the accent. If someone speaks with an accent that we find difficult to understand, it causes us to reduce our verbal interaction with that person because asking a person to repeat what they have said more than once can become embarrassing for both people concerned.

It is the way in which paralinguistics are used that ultimately determines how a message is interpreted and responded to. So if you find yourself walking away from an interaction saying something like: 'I don't know why he got so annoyed, I only asked him to turn the television down, it was irritating everyone!' The reason the man was annoyed was probably to do with the way he was asked to turn down the television. Most people are reasonable and if spoken to respectfully can deal with what they hear very well. It is when the message is delivered in an authoritative, aggressive or hostile tone that communication goes wrong and if accompanied by a different tone, the same message would seem innocuous to most people. The appropriate and effective use of paralinguistics requires awareness of how one uses the tone and pitch of their voice when speaking. Practice in using a calm and even tone with moderate pitch is also required. This does not mean that good communication requires a calm, even and moderate tone all the time but it does mean that when appropriate, it can be used well and effectively and purposefully.

Empathy

> The ability to perceive and reason as well as the ability to communicate understanding of the other person's feelings and their attached meanings. (Reynolds and Scott, 2000, p. 226)

Empathy is a prerequisite for high quality nursing practice because it is fundamental to all helping relationships and the achievement of the goals of clinical nursing (Morse *et al.*, 1992; Peplau, 1997; Reynolds and Scott, 2000). These goals include the need to understand patient distress and to provide supportive interpersonal communication. If nurses fail to empathize with their patients, then they cannot help them to understand or cope effectively as individuals with their illness (Morse *et al.*, 1992, Peplau, 1997, Reynolds and Scott, 2000). Patients value empathetic communication skills such as understanding and anticipation of their needs (McCabe, 2004; Milburn *et al.*, 1995). However, empathy in nursing is a concept that remains poorly understood and its impact on patient outcomes is unclear (Kunyk, 2001; Morse *et al.*, 1992; Reynolds and Scott, 2000). The reason for this could be the traditional association between empathy, in particular 'therapeutic empathy' and the counselling profession. Therapeutic empathy, which is 'a learned communication skill comprised primarily of cognitive and behavioral components which is used to convey understanding of the patients reality', is inappropriate because its purpose is to enable the sufferer to gain insight (Morse *et al.*, 1992, p. 810). However this conceptualization of empathy is primarily that of professional counsellors but is accepted in nursing without question as the central helping component in nurse–patient interaction. That does not mean that nurses should not use therapeutic empathy. Nurses use aspects of counselling skills in their work on a daily basis but they are not counsellors unless they have a specific counselling qualification and the nurse–patient relationship is recognized formally as a counselling one by the nurse and the patient. The difference between therapeutic communication in nursing and therapeutic communication in counselling and psychotherapy lies not in the communication skills required but in the motivation for using them.

For clarity, the empathy that is suggested for everyday use

in nursing is described as basic (Freshwater, 2003). This does not mean that it is less valuable or less therapeutic than 'therapeutic empathy'. Basic empathy is patient-centred communication and is essential for helping relationships and for establishing rapport and trust. It is particularly appropriate for nursing because most relationships between nurses and patients are transient and brief but yet may be quite intense in that the nurse is often required to reduce levels of anxiety and deal with emotional aspects of people's lives. Basic empathy is achieved through the use of active listening skills, questioning and touch in a patient-centred way.

According to Wiseman (1996) the basic requirements of being empathetic are as follows:

- ability to listen;
- ability to take on another's term of reference (imagine what it is like to be them);
- ability to understand and not judge; and
- ability to communicate that understanding.

As discussed in Chapter 1, according to Morse *et al.*'s (1992) model of 'emotional empathy', therapeutic empathetic communication needs to be patient-centred, reflexive and genuine. Specific responses include pity, sympathy, reflexive reassurance and compassion. Responses such as sharing of 'self', reassurance (informing) and therapeutic empathy (learned professional behaviour) are second-level empathy. Non-therapeutic responses include dehumanizing, withdrawing, distancing and labelling.

Morse *et al.* (1992) proposed that communication responses such as sympathy, pity and commiseration have been devalued and labelled unhelpful in nursing and healthcare generally. According to Morse *et al.* (1992) sympathy, which is a first-level empathetic response, is a verbal and non-verbal expression of the nurse's own sorrow or dismay at the patient's situation. When nurses are sympathetic, patients perceive that their feelings of anxiety or distress are justified and value the support from nurses. They find it comforting, reassuring and it can make them feel cared for as an individual. Basic empathetic communication transmits the message of a nurse's understanding and recognition of a patient's situation, it does not mean that nurses are expected to 'fix' or 'solve' all the patient's problems. It is important to note however, that while sympathy, pity and commiseration are valuable empathetic responses, they are part of normal every day communication and within the context of professional practice, a nurse would be required to provide a greater level of emotional help and support to patients when appropriate. Understanding, recognition and support from the nurse are key factors in helping patients cope with their situation themselves. This narrative from McCabe (2004) illustrates this point:

> I think the reassurance from the nurse with me at the time of my diagnosis – that I needed to have an operation . . . she made me feel at ease straight away . . . She just organized everything and was really relaxed and wasn't watching her watch to see was she running late – she was just awfully concerned and at the same time, very professional. She added the human touch, like as if she knew what it was like in my shoes . . . (Claire)

This is a second level empathetic response. The nurse has communicated her understanding of Claire's predicament and is reassuring Claire by sharing her 'self'. Morse *et al.* (1992) describe this type of empathy as 'patient-focused' and it results in patients feeling secure and reassured. Nurses need to value this type of communication for the positive influence it can have on patients but use it in a genuine and patient-centred way. At undergraduate level and when newly qualified, high level empathetic responses can be difficult and perhaps are not required anyway unless a nurse has the necessary counselling qualifications. What is important is that the nurse is supportive and helpful and can recognize the point when a patient may need to be referred to a counsellor, psychologist or psychiatrist as appropriate.

Key points

▶ Communication can be verbal, non-verbal or both.
▶ Communication skills such as, active listening, questioning, touch, paraphrasing and paralinguistics are core skills that can be developed and used in many different ways in any context.

▶ The development of these core communication skills is essential for therapeutic and patient-centred communication requires motivation and practice on the part of the nurse.

▶ Nurses need to develop awareness about how they use core communication skills and the influence this has on the nurse–patient relationship.

▶ Empathy is an important communication skill for nurses and is an integral skill in developing a therapeutic relationship with patients.

▶ A key aspect of the nurse's role is knowing the limitations of their communication skills and referring the patient to an appropriately skilled person, for example a counsellor or psychologist if necessary.

5 Barriers to therapeutic communication

Introduction

As highlighted in previous chapters, one fundamental value that should underpin today's nursing practice is the development of a therapeutic relationship between nurse and patient. Increased patient turnover and shorter hospital stays can militate against the development of a relationship, as can the routine nature of many care interventions that can render the service merely a sequence of tasks, thus jeopardizing the potential for a therapeutic relationship to occur. In addition to the environment, specific communication barriers can exist within the nurse and patient that affect therapeutic communication. Nurse and patient come to the health care situation with their own goals and requirements. Communication facilitates a relationship where these goals merge to form mutual goals (Arnold and Undermann Boggs, 1999). Barriers that exist affect the ability for mutually agreed goals to be achieved.

Thoughtful, insightful and deliberate focus on the therapeutic relationship by nurses serves to enrich the hospital experience for patients (McCabe, 2004; O'Brien, 2000). In a cost- and quality-driven era, the essential and fundamental tasks that relate to the management of each patient may form the priority of care. However, the extension of the nurse's role beyond these tasks, serves to address patients' needs in a more meaningful way.

Specific communication skills outlined in Chapter 4 including non-verbal communication skills (listening and touch) and verbal skills (questioning, information giving and paralinguistics), developing rapport and empathy, are essential building blocks of the therapeutic relationship. However, there are many barriers that exist to the effective use of these skills in the practice setting.

This chapter seeks to understand how barriers in interpersonal relationships, in the context of the therapeutic nurse–patient relationship, affect the quality of a patient's experience. A brief description of the therapeutic relationship in the context of the unique challenges and barriers to communication is outlined. The main barriers that emerge from the literature are explored under the headings barriers in the nurse, barriers in the patient and barriers in the environment. The conclusion includes a reflection on the current literature and highlights how barriers to interpersonal communication can be overcome.

Barriers to the therapeutic relationship

As highlighted in Chapter 3, Peplau's (1952, 1991) work resolutely emphasized the interpersonal nature of nursing as contributing to the distinctive role that nursing can offer to health care (Aggleton and Chalmers, 2000). Peplau (1952, 1991) introduced the idea of the therapeutic relationship as being a human connection that heals. Similarly, the influence of theory principles from other disciplines such as Freud (Dworetzky, 1997); Buber's (1958) I–Thou relationship; Rogers' (1961) humanistic approach and Maslow's (1954) stages of self-development all served to influence the proposal that nursing care should be patient-centred (Arnold and Undermann Boggs, 1999). It is only through good communication skills identified in Chapter 4, and the development of the therapeutic relationship (Chapter 3) that nurses can truly identify and respond to the unique needs of their patients in a patient-centred way. Howard-Harwood (1997) suggested that the establishment of this relationship is essential to the provision of a truly safe environment for the patient.

Communication is valued as a fundamental nursing role. Good communication is at the core of the therapeutic relationship that nurses strive to attain with patients in their care. Inadequate use of communication skills presents a barrier to the development of a therapeutic relationship (Keating *et al.*, 2002). Costa (2001) recommended that nurses develop specific *therapeutic* communication skills in order to address patients' needs more fully. This included being 'truly present' to the patient, manifested by being able to listen; being perceptive to the environment; and being able to anticipate patients' needs. These communication skills were deemed fundamental to the therapeutic relationship: being able to identify individual informational needs, empowering patients and being present to patients (Costa, 2001; James, 2000; Mitchell, 1997; Otte, 1996). However barriers exist to the operation of these skills in practice. These can occur within the nurse, within the patient and within the environment.

Barriers in the nurse

Keating *et al.* (2002) examined barriers to nurse–patient relationships and suggested an urgent need for improvement of communication skills. In a pilot study in Australia 199 nurses and 36 consumers participated in 14 workshops to provide data. It was found that communication was identified as the principal barrier to the development of the relationship. Keating *et al.* (2002) found that the reported listening skills of nurses in the study featured as the most prominent barrier to communication and relationship development.

Crotty (1985), Hodges *et al.* (1986) and Reid (1985) highlighted that nurses often did not communicate well with patients, and approached patients only to deal with administrative or functional activities. This is echoed within mental health settings (O Brien 2000) and indeed 'lack of communication' was an emerging theme in McCabe's (2004) study of patients' communication experiences within an acute general hospital. The participants in this latter study frequently referred to nurses not providing enough information and many commented on how nurses were more concerned with tasks rather than with talking with them. However, all the participants felt that it was not the nurses' fault as they were too 'busy'.

Bergen (1992), Haggman-Laitila and Astedt-Kurki (1994), Hostutler *et al.* (1999), Jarman (1995) and Jarrett and Payne (2000) all suggested that nurses may undervalue communication in the health care setting and that they may be unaware of the meaning and significance of the nurse–patient relationship for patients. This lack of awareness by nurses results in them making assumptions about what nursing care a patient needs or wants because, often, they do not ask patients (Bergen, 1992, Booth *et al.*, 1996; McCabe, 2004). Active listening is essential in patient-centred communication, however barriers to listening exist in the health care context.

Listening

As indicated in Chapter 4, good listening skills are essential requisites of nursing. Markanday (1997) stated that every patient is an unique individual and should collaborate in the planning of his own care, which can only be facilitated through listening to patients' needs. Inadequate listening skills can result in patient confusion and anxiety (Otte, 1996). Phillips (1992) suggested that good listening skills also help prevent mistakes from occurring. Poor listening skills were uncovered by Costa's (2001) study. One nurse casually dismissed a patient who expressed a fear of dying during surgery. Clearly, the item was heard but the patient's real feelings, fears and needs in this particular area were not attended to. Albeit one situation, this highlights clearly the major omissions that can occur if active listening is not carried out. Gibbons (1993) suggested that nurses find it difficult to listen because their work is so action-oriented.

Using listening skills in conjunction with questioning skills and observing patient cues, allows the nurse to operate truly patient-centred communication. Within all individuals barriers exist to listening such as a preoccupation with what one wishes to say next, or self-consciousness (Sidell, 2000). This latter element is a preoccupation with oneself during the communication, thus precipitating thoughts about the next job to be done, for example. This can deflect from the focus on the individual who is actually talking. Other recognized barriers include stress, anxiety, poor attention, misinterpretations and the use of 'rehearsing responses' (Burnard, 1997). While generalized barriers to effective listening are common, nurses and other health care workers have an unique responsibility to listen to patients to ascertain patient reactions, questions, needs and problems. It is essential that *active* listening take place. This is where the nurse makes a deliberate and conscious effort to listen to the patient, hear and recognize what is being said and plan care accordingly.

Active listening is not an automatic passive behaviour. True active listening involves more than just hearing (Burnard, 1997). It involves a range of behaviours, such as using prompts or phrases – to encourage the other person – to a variety of non-verbal behaviours. It involves reflection upon what is being said and understanding the person's perspective. Therefore, it is both a cognitive and an emotional process (Arnold and Underman Boggs, 1999).

Barriers to active listening may result from a failure to fully engage with the patient. While the nurse may appear to be listening, adjunct non-verbal behaviours that support active listening (including the use of appropriate body posture and gestures by the nurse) may give conflicting messages. In McCabe's (2004) study the nurses gave an impression of being busy through non-verbal means. It was communicated clearly (although not verbally) to all of these patients that the nurse was too busy to talk. A failure to align oneself opposite and proximal to the patient (sitting or standing), provide appropriate venue or time, absence of interested facial expression, nodding of the head, and lack of open posture (Sidell, 2000) may all demonstrate that the nurse is not paying attention (Burnard, 1997) to what the patient has to say. There is failure to attend.

 Exercise

Without explaining the exercise, ask a friend or partner to tell you about their last holiday. Listen, but while you are listening avoid non-verbal gestures such as nodding, smiling and interested facial expression. Also, sit in a way that avoids an 'open posture' (arms and legs crossed, not facing the person). Ask for feedback on you as a listener. You will be surprised at the barriers created by your lack attention and feedback using non-verbal cues.

Nurses keen to improve their listening skills can practise sitting directly opposite the patient who is also seated, maintaining a relaxed 'open' body position, leaning slightly towards the patient and maintaining good eye contact (Burnard, 1997). It is also important in a busy, rushed environment, to give time, or at least the perception of time for the patient. Rather than appearing busy or action-orientated as described by Gibbons (1993) the use of attending skills when listening increases the likelihood of reducing barriers that exist. Attending behaviour was described as the physical demonstration of nurses' accessibility and readiness to listen to patients through the use of non-verbal communication (Stein-Parbury, 1993).

Attending is a skill that is valued highly by patients. Indeed it was an emerging theme in McCabe's (2004) study. Although the participants of this study did not refer directly to the term 'attending', they described nursing behaviours they valued which were specific to attending. These behaviours were elucidated as 'giving time and being there', 'open/honest communication' and 'genuineness'. 'Being there' was also an emergent theme in O'Brien's (2000) study. In O'Brien's study being present to patients emerged strongly from the data. In addition to its function within attending, the *presence* of the nurses in studies (Costa, 2001; McCabe, 2004; O'Brien, 2000) involved self-disclosure, genuineness and empathy. This empathetic understanding, as Corbett (2001) described it, is a special dimension in the building of a caring relationship, which fundamentally comprises of acceptance and respect without prejudice and also without any inference of agreement or disagreement, approval or disapproval, simply to perceive the world as the patient does. These skills are also central to the caring role of the nurse (Corbett, 2001), which is considered fundamental to nursing (Pearson *et al.*, 2000).

Barriers exist to specific areas of non-verbal communication such as touch.

Touch

Touch is a highly valued non-verbal communication in nursing (DeVos, 1989; Nesbitt Blondis and Jackson, 1982; Wondrak,

1998). However, there are barriers to its use within nursing. In one study, out of 149 touches observed only seven were deemed to be of an expressive nature (McCann and McKenna, 1993). Similarly in Routasalo's (1996) study just under half of the 196 touches were associated with tasks. Although nurses frequently pat the patient on the arms, shoulders, hair and forehead (Oliver and Redfern, 1991), touch associated with nursing tasks takes precedence.

Because of the potential intimacy of physical touch there are further barriers to its use in practice. Although the nurse may reassure or greet a patient with a pat on the hand, hand-hold, or touch to the shoulder, this may cause discomfort for either the client or the nurse for a variety of personal reasons (Gleeson and Timmins, 2004). Patients can feel uncomfortable with touch (McCann and McKenna, 1993) particularly touching of the face, or placing an arm around a shoulder. According to the McCann and McKenna (1993) study, elderly male patients expressed concerns about male nurses touching them as it conveyed feelings of homosexuality. In Edwards' (1998) study one male patient stated that it 'did not feel right having a male nurse doing such intimate tasks'.

Knowledge and awareness of these barriers are essential to the skilful use of touch. In addition, touching should not be provided to patients in a routine way. Patient preference and need should be identified. It should be confined in most situations to patting or holding the hand.

Barriers can also exist within the nurse with regard to verbal communication particularly in relation to language.

Language

Nurses have a responsibility to give vital information to patients to facilitate their recovery. Non-adherence with prescribed measures can occur if the message is not communicated effectively. Morrall (2001) found that the use of professional jargon could contribute to non-adherence to a treatment regimen. Indeed, overuse of specialist language was recognized as a potential barrier to communication as it serves to alienate the patient (Sidell, 2000). O'Shea (2004) found that doctors often provided information that parents did not understand and required translation and simplification by nurses after the event.

Factors that can improve the effectiveness of the health care message include simplifying the information being given, the use of repetition to reinforce the message and being specific. It is imperative that communication is clear and easily understood (Otte, 1996). This should all be delivered, in as much as is possible or feasible, in an individual manner, directed towards each new patient, thus avoiding the lack of individuality experienced by patients in Costa's (2001) study. Written information has also been shown to increase knowledge, improve compliance and improve outcome (Ogden, 2000). A significant barrier to effective communication is lack of nurse skills to support people with hearing loss, or who have very limited English. Therapeutic relationships should identify the need for specifically trained personnel and use of appropriate responsive written information (Wood and Alligood, 2002).

Patients who do not speak the native language of a country face additional barriers to engaging effectively in communication. Poor communication between non-English speaking Somali women and health workers was identified as a problem in Davies and Bath's (2001) study, and restricted women's information seeking behaviour. Even though interpreters were provided, fears about misinterpretation and confidentiality restricted the women's use of this service.

The presence and use of written instructions and information leaflets in a variety of pertinent languages can be useful to overcome the language barrier. However, it is important that these are developed with the patient in mind and avoid overuse of sophisticated language. The patient's ethnic origin and previous experience of reading are also crucial. Illiteracy is an identified barrier to learning, and with much communication relying upon written materials; it can cause problems for the patient (Doak et al., 1985). Even where there is no illiteracy as such, many educational reading materials are written at a level that presents reading difficultly to the average patient (Zion and Aiman, 1989). An accurate assessment of the patient's reading ability is required to ensure that these learning tools are useful. However, this is not always possible, as patients may not admit to a reading deficit. It is important, therefore, that nursing staff back up written information with verbal and non-verbal information and involve members of the family in teaching sessions.

Other barriers that can occur within individual nurses are communication filters.

Comunication filters

Hindle (2003) referred to aspects of individuals that distort the receipt of the communication message as 'filters'. He described these as: defence mechanisms; attitudes, beliefs and values; prejudices; and perceptual disturbances. These can adversely affect communication in the health care setting.

As described in Chapter 3, Freud introduced the concepts of transference and counter-transference. Transference occurs when individuals unconsciously project seemingly inappropriate or irrational feelings/attitudes towards others that are based on previous personal experiences. Counter-transference refers to the nurse's unconscious or conscious response to the patient based on the patient's irrational feelings/attitudes towards them or their own biases, beliefs and values (Gallop and O'Brien, 2003; O'Kelly, 1998). Over-involvement and withdrawal are expressions of counter-transference in the nurse's behaviour (O'Kelly, 1998). Defence mechanisms were also described by Freud, and commonly accepted as patterns of human behaviour (Hindle, 2003). These include rationalization (defending behaviour with reasons that may be illegitimate), regression (reverting to behaviour associated with childhood), repression (suppressing emotions), denial (refusing to accept events), identification (taking on the characteristics of another) and projection (projecting one's own undesirable traits onto another). These behaviours may be present in either the patient or the nurse (or both) and can impair perception of communication thus affecting the development of a therapeutic relationship. For example:

One of your nursing colleagues expresses disgust that a patient is a smoker, yet she is a smoker herself (projection).

A colleague is repeatedly late for work and has a repertoire of plausible excuses without accepting her responsibility for her own tardiness (rationalization).

Both of the above examples demonstrate that the presence of these 'filters' hampers the open, honest communication that patients desire (McCabe, 2004) and which are essential to good communication and the therapeutic relationship. While an acceptance and understanding of these defence mechanisms in patients is required by nurses, their presence in nurses needs to be explored through self-awareness and personal development (see Chapter 9) in order for the nurse to function effectively in the health care setting.

Other psychological factors influencing communication are attitudes, values and beliefs (Hindle, 2003). The beliefs of the nurse in Edwards' (1998) study (she considered the patient's touch to be sexual) directly affected her behaviour towards that patient (anger). Similarly, touch practices in general appeared to be strongly influenced by attitudes, values and beliefs originating within the nurse's own family of origin. According to Northouse and Northouse (1998) some individuals are born into families where there is an enormous amount of touching. On the other hand some individuals are raised in families where touch is limited only to task situations. Thus personal attitudes, beliefs and values can have a powerful influence on communication behaviour by nurses and through increasing self-awareness and personal development, skills can be aligned with good communication practice. In general, nurses need to be aware of their potential defence mechanisms and set these aside in their interactions with patients. Thus nurses can be accepting, open, honest and genuine in that relationship and utilize effective listening and attending skills to support their verbal skills. Similarly, attitudes, beliefs and values that are negative need to recognized and set aside in the nurse–patient interaction, and replaced, where possible, with those that are more positive. This can be done through exploring attitudes, beliefs and values, reading nursing literature and researching the area, developing an increased understanding of the patient situation and aligning beliefs accordingly.

Prejudices were another psychological factor identified by Hindle (2003) that can affect nurse–patient communication. Prejudice involves 'making assumptions about people and attributing certain labels and stereotypes to them' (Hindle, 2003, p. 62). Kirkham *et al.* (2002) described the use of stereotyping as a defence mechanism by midwives to cope with their professional role. They found that midwives sometimes misjudged women's ability and willingness to participate in their maternity care and, as a consequence, women were negatively labelled, for example, as demanding and/or as uncooperative. Midwives often formulated their opinions about their clients on the basis of circumstances over which childbearing women exercised little control: housing tenure, age and/or social class. Even when such judgements were shown to be erroneous, they generally endured throughout the maternity episode. They suggest that stereotyping by nurses, although possibly a 'coping mechanism in the face of limited resources' was 'corrosive' in that it affected the therapeutic relationship, particularly in relation to choice and decision making.

Similarly, Somali women in Davies and Bath's (2001) study perceived that they were denied information due to punitive attitudes and prejudiced views among health professionals. Likewise, Bowler (1993) investigated the delivery of maternity care to women of South Asian decent in Britain using an ethnographic approach. She found that the midwives commonly held stereotypical views of women. Their stereotype of women of Asian descent contained four main themes: communication problems; failure to comply with care and service abuse; making a fuss about nothing; and a lack of normal maternal instinct. Equally, Green *et al.* (1990) in their study of expectant mothers found two commonly encountered stereotypes attributed to women: the 'well educated, middle-class NCT type' and the 'uneducated working class woman'.

Prejudice commonly, although not exclusively, occurs in ethnic minority groups. The older person may also encounter this (Williams *et al.*, 2004) whereby assumptions are made about hospitalized older people (that they are cognitively impaired and require 'baby talk' as a form of communication). Similarly those with mental illness may also experience prejudice. A study conducted in Durban, South Africa, found that 90 per cent of the nurses in a general hospital setting held negative attitudes toward people with mental illnesses (Mavundla and Uys, 1997). Jorm *et al.* (1999) reported that health professionals were more likely to discriminate against those with mental illness, compared with the general public. Similarly, Foster and Onyeukwu (2003) reported negative attitudes in forensic nurses towards substance misuse in the mentally ill. Prejudice can also exist towards those whose sexual orientation differs from that of the nurse, although attitudes towards lesbians and gay men do appear to be more positive than previously reported (Röndahl *et al.*, 2004). Similarly, those experiencing certain illness such as HIV/AIDS can experience prejudice (Cree *et al.*, 2004). Negative attitudes and prejudice related to HIV/AIDS also occurs among health professionals (Valimaki *et al.*, 1998).

Thomas and Dines (1994) suggested that as professionals working in a multicultural society nurses and midwives ought to be able to respond to these needs appropriately. Great care must be taken to explore and reflect upon personal attitudes and behaviour when nursing these patients. Through self-awareness and personal development (Chapter 9) these issues can be addressed. This is important because these can form significant barriers to communication in the health care context and to the overall aim of developing a therapeutic relationship with patients. Developing an empathetic understanding of individuals may help to overcome this. Listening skills can also be improved through self-awareness and personal development. Seeking educational opportunities is also important.

The nurse is but one aspect of the nurse–patient relationship and barriers also exist with respect to patients.

Barriers within patients

Unequal power relationships

Earlier in the chapter we discussed the variety of responses that patients may have to the use of touch and cautioned against routine use without first establishing patients' views and needs within the context of the therapeutic relationship. This area reveals patient vulnerability with regard to communication. Edwards (1998) found that while in hospital, patients often expect to be touched. This may be attributed to the depersonalization and subordination of patients as individuals while in care.

Edward's (1998) notion of the subordinate patient in the nurse–patient touch scenario needs to be borne in mind in the nursing situation. In many clinical situations, the power base often rests with the health care workers, and not the patient. Touch can be perceived as a manifestation of that power (Northouse and Northouse, 1998). Routasalo (1996) found that typically touch was nurse initiated and occurred when the nurse was in a standing position while the patient was sitting or lying down in bed. Patients in a health care setting expect to be touched, and nurses, perceiving this to be a caring gesture, may touch individuals in ways ordinarily reserved for close family. Patients can interpret this in a negative way, conceiving it to be condescending (Hollinger and Buschmann, 1993).

These issues identify potentially important barriers to effective communication in the health care setting. Morrall (2003) described the social factors affecting communication under the headings freedom, power, sickness and social discourse. Much of this discussion resonates the emergent findings from the literature regarding touch. The relationship with a patient who is a health care recipient is socially constructed and the patient may be in a dependent role by virtue of their patient status. As demonstrated in many of the studies, patients may receive a pat on the head, whether they like it or not, and sometimes they don't! Thus indicating the effect of the social construction of healthcare in some settings where patients are not equal partners in decisions affecting their care. Likewise the potential power exerted by nurses is evidenced in its use for persuasion purposes (Edwards 1998). Furthermore the 'sick role' that Morrall (2003) described may contribute to the patient's acceptance of touch as part of the health care experience.

The potential construction of unequal power relationships, the social construction of health and illness and the potential sick role can all potentially affect communication within the health care setting (Morrall, 2003). The likely effect of these experiences is that the patient may not be able to engage fully in a therapeutic relationship due to their perceived dependence and lack of autonomy. They may not act as equal partners in their care and become passive recipients of care. These types of barriers contribute to the wider notion of environmental barriers.

Environmental barriers

There are environmental barriers to using communication skills and patient-centred communication at a practice level (Rogan-Foy and Timmins, 2004). These concern the failure to individualize nursing care and ritualistic nursing actions.

Failure to individualize nursing care

A predominant theme in Costa's (2001) phenomenological study of 16 patients who had undergone day surgery was 'not being recognized as individuals'. Respondents in this study recognized and acknowledged the presence of the nurse as valuable to their recovery, thus indicating the therapeutic potential of the nurse role itself. Costa (2001) recommended that nurses needed to develop specific therapeutic communication skills including, being 'truly present' to the patient, manifested by being able to listen, being perceptive to the environment and being able to anticipate patients' needs.

Ritualistic nursing action

Nursing has long been associated with the use of rituals and tradition, and although these have declined in many areas of nursing they still prevail (Jacobson, 2000; Riegel *et al.*, 1996; Strange, 2001). This use of ritual affects the nurse's ability to communicate effectively (Martin, 1998). Rather than an open communication system Martin (1998) suggested that communication rituals are socially constructed within the healthcare setting, and communication during nursing procedures is often condensed and restricted and ultimately a source of patient control, rather than a therapeutic intervention.

Martin (1998) attributed nurses' use of rituals to what he termed ' professional distancing', whereby; perhaps due to the emotional burden of care, nurses distance themselves from the patients. This distancing has obvious repercussions for nurse–patient communication. The nature of ritualistic communication is unlikely to be patient-centred as it serves the purpose of the nurse. Rituals, Martin (1998) proposed, were also bound in 'task orientation'. Despite a rhetoric of patient-centred care, the focus of many hospital wards is on getting the work done (Martin, 1998). He suggests that this contributes to the 'busy nurse' syndrome which keeps the nurse active all the time and protects him/her from the need to talk to the patient. This busyness allows the nurse to 'legitimately distance themselves from patients' thus allowing 'no time for nurse–patient interaction' (Martin, 1998). Patients in McCabe's (2004) study identified busyness as a legitimate reason for the lack of communication by nurses. This has obvious potential repercussions for nurse–patient communication. We need to consider how to overcome these potential barriers.

Overcoming barriers

It is essential that nurses explore current methods of communication delivery, existent barriers and methods for overcoming these, particularly in the presence of additional barriers such as language and hearing loss. Communication and the therapeutic nurse–patient relationship situation is not an esoteric element of nursing, but rather a fundamental aspect of caring. It is within this context that improvements in this area need to be considered. Areas that may be considered include family involvement, nursing theory and conceptual model use. Developing self-awareness and using reflection are other tools to identify and deal with barriers to communication and these are explored in Chapters 9 and 10.

Family involvement

The therapeutic relationship, partnership and empowerment are not confined entirely to the patient. The client does not live in the world in isolation, but rather as a part of a family, community and environment. It is increasingly being recognized that the social support has an important role in the health care dynamic between patient and nurse, and in the past this vital aspect of the patient has been overlooked in many settings. The diversity of the patient's social support needs acceptance and identification in the health care context. Social support from others outside the health care setting is a perceived source of comfort for patients (Ogden, 2000). A sense of comfort was noted from previous studies of day surgery by the presence of family members both pre-operatively and post-operatively, and showed a significant effect on the patient's perceived sense of social support (Costa, 2001; Mitchell, 1997; Ogden, 2000). Driscoll (2000) also found that the inclusion of carers when information is given to patients improved the level of satisfaction with information given thus reducing the carers' anxiety after discharge and also decreased the possibility of experiencing any medical problems at home. Simons and Robertson (2002) found that parents were in a good position to act as advocates for their children. The obvious benefits from family involvement need to be incorporated into practice. Allowing the attendance of some family members where possible may be a source of comfort and facilities for this should be provided. At a more fundamental level, the vital communication skills that are fundamental to the therapeutic relationship need to be extended to the family to provide a holistic approach to care.

Education

There is no substitute, however, for education and training, which is known to improve communication skills. Indeed, Chambers-Evans *et al.* (1999) found that the experience gained by nurses participating in a qualitative research interview training project helped them to obtain a deeper understanding of nurse–patient communication by utilizing skills such as listening, understanding and validating responses. It is imperative, therefore, that nurses and employers explore communication training options available to them. Betts (2003) identified education as crucial to improving nurses' communication skills and highlighted a deficit in skills training among nurses.

Keating *et al.* (2002), who identified barriers to nurse–patient relationships among 119 nurses in Australia, found that communication was identified as the principal barrier to the development of the relationship.

Education can have a positive effect on the communication skills of nurses (Chambers-Evans *et al.*, 1999). However, the lack of good communication suggests the need for a holistic framework to guide and direct nursing practice in this area (Betts, 2003). From a systematic review of the literature Michie *et al.* (2003) identified the ability to elicit and discuss patients' beliefs and the ability to activate the patient to take control as integral components of such a model. Similarly, Fossum and Arborelius (2004) found from an observation study of outpatient doctor/patient interactions that involving the patient in management led to more successful communication. Fossum and Arborelius (2004) also amalgamated the findings of previous studies into suggestions to improve patient-centred communication. These recommendations included:

● providing the opportunity for patients to express their needs, including symptoms, thoughts, feelings and expectations;
● treating the patient as a person with a health need, rather than the perception of the person as a disease entity; and
● ensuring that the patient feels that they have been understood.

Gallant *et al.* (2002) reiterated that clients often develop sophisticated knowledge about how to manage their illness. It has been found that consumers of health care value the process of shared decision-making whereby they feel respected and make a meaningful contribution to the discussions as well as clear arrangements for review of the treatment decisions (Edwards *et al.*, 2003).

It is from this perspective that the concept of partnership can be introduced into the modern health care system as a way of overcoming barriers to communication. The therapeutic relationship fulfils the criteria of a partnership as it reflects an interpersonal relationship between two or more people towards mutually defined goals (Gallant *et al.*, 2002). The roles and responsibilities of the partners may vary during this partnership; in essence the nurse promotes client empowerment and competency by sustaining the relationship and reinforcing client progress, supporting decision making and assisting the client to develop more knowledge and skills (Gallant *et al.*, 2002).

Nursing theory and conceptual model use

Nursing theory and conceptual model use as described in Chapter 2, also provide a way forward for overcoming barriers to communication in the practice setting. Partnership in the nurse–patient relationship with a recognition of patient autonomy is a recurring theme throughout popular nursing theory (Pearson *et al.*, 2000). The development of a nurse–patient relationship was a fundamental component of Peplau's (1952, 1991) work. This particular aspect of nursing has particular relevance for moving away from the medical, traditional and routine models of care (Pearson *et al.*, 2000).

Lack of individualization of care is a barrier to communication and inability to individualize, resulting in care of women based upon stereotypes, emerged in Bowler's (1993) study. Conceptual models have contributed much to the individualization of nursing (Tierney, 1998). Roper *et al.* (2001) emphasized the individual nature of this process of nursing and the necessity for patient participation, all elements of what we may begin to consider as patient-centred care. Their model also allows for specific assessment of individual needs and problems in the activity of living (AL), and thus may be said to facilitate patient-centred communication.

Partnership is an explicit aspect of the use of the SCDNT as a conceptual model in practice (Orem, 2001). Empowerment is also crucial. Rather than nursing care being regarded solely as providing direct care to another, Orem (2001) also highlighted the important nursing actions of supporting and educating patients. The development of the nurse–patient relationship was identified as crucial to this process (Orem, 2001) as it is essential for the full and participative involvement of patients in care as suggested.

The identified barriers that exist may be also be related to an underpinning lack of communication skills. One of the fundamental values that should underpin today's nursing practice is the development of a therapeutic relationship between nurse and patient (Arnold and Undermann Boggs, 1999). This relationship is emphasized throughout the literature on the topic (Aggleton and Chalmers, 2000; Howard-Harwood, 1997). It is only through good communication, and the development of the therapeutic relationship that nurses can truly identify the unique needs of their patients and address potential barriers that may exist. This process underpins contemporary approaches to communication within health care settings (Ito and Lambert, 2002) and supports a nurse–patient communication that is patient-centred.

In today's accelerated health care environment, where cost and quality issues predominate; we must not lose sight of the fundamental communication skills required by nurses. At the heart of nursing is caring. Recent studies indicate the high value that patients place on the presence of the nurse. It is essential that nurses value their own unique contribution to the health care setting, and through personal awareness, reflect and build upon their communication skills. It is only through the provision of a relationship where the nurse can listen to patients and address their unique needs that quality care can be implemented.

Key points

▶ Many barriers exist to the effective development and use of core communication skills in nursing. These barriers can be within the nurse, within the patient or within the environment.

▶ Barriers within the nurse include: lack of communication skills, undervaluing communication as an integral part of nursing and a lack of awareness of the meaning and significance of nurse–patient communication in providing high quality patient-centred care.

▶ A nurse's personal values, beliefs, attitudes and prejudices can adversely affect the nurse–patient relationship.

▶ Patient-centredness and shared decision making are regarded as key factors in preventing barriers to effective and positive communication.

6 Communicating in difficult situations

Introduction

Some situations are seen by students to be 'difficult' due to the emotional content, perceived lack of communication ability and cultural differences. These situations pose a significant challenge for personal and professional development. They can involve a combination of interaction with patients, their relatives and colleagues; and learning to communicate in an effective and patient- or person-centred way in these situations is essential for developing confidence and positive relationships. However, students often feel that although the theory delivered in the class setting is relevant, it does not prepare them for the reality of dealing with these situations. In this chapter we hope to help students meet these challenges by providing theory in relation to dealing with issues such as breaking bad news, anxiety, hostility and cultural differences. In conjunction with this theory we will demonstrate to students that by learning to manage themselves in difficult situations rather than trying to manage others who may be emotionally distressed or poor communicators themselves, a much more positive and patient- or person-centred outcome can be achieved.

Although this chapter will deal specifically with the difficult issues associated with breaking bad news, cultural issues and anxiety and hostility, it is important to acknowledge that the situations that individuals perceive as difficult vary greatly from person to person. This is primarily because of their existing communication skills, their level of self-confidence and their past experiences in relation to a particular situation. For example, some nurses may find it more difficult to approach their manager to request study leave or annual leave, than helping a patient who has received bad news or helping a recently bereaved family.

If nurses perceive that they do not have the communication skills needed to communicate effectively in 'difficult' situations they may avoid them or they may communicate in a negative or unhelpful way. This can have an adverse affect on a nurse's level of confidence and overall professional development. Also if a nurse avoids dealing with very emotive situations, patients can feel very lonely and isolated because the nurse does not acknowledge or talk about what is happening to the patient. It is, therefore, essential that the communication skills required for dealing successfully and appropriately with difficult situations are recognized, developed and practised by nurses.

One of the most effective learning opportunities for students to see how certain communication skills can help in difficult situations is to identify a role model. Identify a nurse who is known to be a good communicator; that is, kind, sympathetic, non-judgemental, open and friendly. With these characteristics and experience he or she will probably also be empathetic. You can usually identify these nurses from your own experiences with them or through observing how they have very positive relationships with patients and colleagues. If a nurse is kind, supportive and helpful towards students, then it is probably fair to say that they are the same towards patients and their colleagues and would be, therefore, a good role model. In addition to using a good or positive role model it is also helpful to identify a nurse whose communication skills are not as positive and observe how poor communication skills impact on the nurse–patient relationship and patient care generally.

Managing yourself in difficult situations

As mentioned earlier, it is important that a nurse learns to manage himself/herself in difficult situations. If they are unable to do this or are not aware of their skills and behaviours then they will find it difficult to build confidence in approaching difficult situations and dealing with them effectively. This section talks about the need to know yourself and the assumptions, values, beliefs and attitudes that you hold that influence your approach toward people both socially and in your work. If you feel this is an aspect of yourself that you have not thought much about then it might be beneficial for you to read Chapter 9, which deals with the role of self-concept, self-awareness and self-esteem in personal and professional development, before completing this chapter. By identifying our hidden assumptions, values, beliefs and attitudes it is possible to interpret situations that we perceive to be difficult in a more accurate way. When this happens the action that we take can be more patient-centred and helpful. Our reaction to situations that were previously perceived as difficult is now more manageable and less stressful.

A nurse is in the process of admitting a very elderly lady to an acute medical ward. The lady appears to be confused, is agitated and has a raised body temperature. Her personal hygiene is very poor and she is very thin. Her next of kin is documented as her daughter who lives with her and brought her to hospital. She has gone home to bring in some clothes, shoes and other personal belongings for her mother. The nurse discusses this patient with a nursing colleague and voices her annoyance with the lady's daughter because the lady is so physically unwell and unkempt. The nurse's irritation grows as it takes a number of hours for the patient's daughter to return to the hospital with her mother's belongings. When the nurse enters the patient's room she sees the daughter sitting in a chair beside her mother's bed. With an irritated tone and loud voice the nurse asks the daughter to give her some details for the nursing notes regarding her mother's illness and medical history. The daughter begins to tell the nurse how her father, the patient's husband, died four weeks previously and he was the main carer for her mother who had been in bad health for a number of years. The nurse's facial expression shows her further irritation as her continuous cold tone asks why the patient's condition deteriorated so rapidly and why she did not come to hospital sooner. The daughter then becomes upset and tells the nurse that she herself has poor health and although she tried to look after her mother she could not manage. When the nurse asks her why she could not manage the daughter becomes even more distressed and shows her hands and wrists that are grossly deformed as a result of chronic arthritis. The nurse is immediately sympathetic and her attitude towards the patient and her mother changes to a more sensitive and supportive approach.

This example describes how ordinary everyday events at work can become stressful or negative. This example highlights how hidden assumptions can make interpretations of situations inaccurate and reactions negative. It also supports the discussion in Chapter 4 that suggests asking questions starting with 'why' can be judgemental, whereas questions using 'what' or 'how' can provide more specific, focused answers that are less judgemental or difficult to answer. The thing about our assumptions, values, beliefs and attitudes is that they exist sometimes within our consciousness but often outside our consciousness. What we need to do to manage ourselves in difficult situations is to identify them so that we can change or ignore our assumptions, values, beliefs and attitudes in order to focus on the needs of patients in many different contexts.

Anxiety also plays a key role in how a nurse communicates with a patient and can make some situations difficult for both the nurse and the patient. Anxiety is an emotional response that represents feelings of discomfort, insecurity or fear. It generally manifests physically as nausea or sweating, and can affect a person's behaviour (Kreigh and Perko, 1983).

The anxiety can be nurse-related, patient-related or both, for example, a nurse may be anxious about removing sutures from a wound because they may hurt the patient or he/she may not have much experience in removing sutures. Likewise the patient may be feeling anxious because he/she thinks the procedure will be painful. Anxiety can trigger hostile or angry responses in people because they are misinterpreting your words. They may not even be aware of their own anxiety and this can make the situation even more difficult and prevent effective communication. Every person whether a patient or family member experiences some level of anxiety when in hospital. This means that when communicating, nurses need to keep this in mind and understand that one person can be as anxious about having heart surgery as another person having a toenail removed. An appreciation of this will help nurses communicate more appropriately and in a patient-centred way when helping patients to identify the possible causes of their anxiety. Kreigh and Perko (1983) refer to anxiety as mild, moderate or severe and describe the effect of anxiety on behaviour and ability to think clearly.

● *Mild anxiety*. Thinking and coping ability is enhanced and behaviours may include walking, humming, restlessness but focused when necessary. A nurse will experience this before carrying out a procedure for the first time, like catheterization or removing sutures.

● *Moderate anxiety*. Concentration and the ability to think clearly is reduced and the person may not know what is making them anxious. They will appear tense and possibly agitated, angry or even withdrawn. They will respond well to support and guidance at this level of anxiety. This level of anxiety is apparent in patients and their relatives when on admission to hospital or just prior to surgery.

● *Severe anxiety*. Cannot think logically or coherently even with guidance. Behaviour is unfocused and possibly inappropriate. Response to support and guidance is not immediate. Referral to a psychologist or psychiatrist is recommended.

Below is an example of how anxiety influences communication:

A young woman is admitted to the emergency department following a road traffic accident. She has a concussion and minor facial lacerations. Shortly afterwards her father arrives in the department and spends some time with her. Then he leaves to go home to get some personal items for his daughter who needs to be admitted, but he returns to the department almost immediately to say that his car has been clamped by hospital parking attendants. He is very irate and the nurse finds it difficult to calm him down. He says that there were no parking places when he arrived and he had to park in a 'no parking' zone. His anxiety about his daughter meant that he felt that the only option was to park illegally. The nurse understands this and asks the man to take a seat beside her while she phones the parking attendant. She explains the situation to the parking attendant who says that the clamp will be removed without charge but that the man will have to wait about 20 minutes. The man complains further when he hears this but the nurse uses this opportunity to talk to him about his daughter's accident and what treatment she will need. Eventually the man starts to tell the nurse about how scared he was driving to the hospital and not knowing what to expect and after a few minutes he thanks the nurse for helping him out and goes to spend more time with his daughter before the clamp is removed from his car.

The following points are useful for ensuring effective communication and helping patients deal with anxiety:

- always appreciate that being admitted to hospital, regardless of the reason, provokes anxiety in patients and their relatives;
- actively address the concerns of the patient or relative. In the above example the nurse deals with the clamping issue before she addresses the main cause of the man's anxiety, which is his daughter and her injuries. Trying to reduce a person's level of anxiety without dealing with their immediate concerns will be ineffective and may only heighten their anxiety;
- ensure privacy when trying to reduce a patient's or relative's anxiety and let them know that you are genuinely concerned for them. Pull the curtains around the bed, sit if possible and look at the patient and relatives when they speak. Active listening is an essential skill in helping people deal with their anxiety. Be honest about the choices a person has or what the situation is and do not make promises you can't keep. Speak slowly and repeat the main points if necessary. Just because you attempt to reduce a person's anxiety level, do not assume that they will respond positively. They may not be ready to talk but by checking on them and keeping them updated with information, patients and their relatives will begin to trust the nurse and this will reduce their anxiety levels;
- be aware of your own levels of anxiety. This will allow you to deal more effectively with the anxieties of others or help you realize that maybe you are not the best person to help. This is important because a key role in nursing is recognizing when a patient needs someone else to help them besides a nurse. A counsellor, psychologist or psychiatrist is often the most appropriate person to help a patient deal with moderate or severe levels of anxiety.

Breaking bad news

Nurses do not usually break bad news to patients directly but are generally, although not always, present when patients and their families are given bad news. A key role of the nurse is to clarify, explain and expand on what the doctor said. However, before we discuss how to do that it is essential to talk about what nurses expect to contribute to family, relatives and friends who have just lost a loved one or to a patient who has just heard that they have a terminal illness or will need to have a leg amputated. The role of the nurse in caring for patients is to provide either physical or psychological comfort and support. However when caring for a bereaved person, nurses can find it difficult to see results of their endeavours to help the other person. Usually they never know if they made any difference to how that person coped when they heard the bad news. Because nurses do not receive feedback from the bereaved person they can assume incorrectly that they did not help sufficiently and many, therefore, try to detach themselves from these situations. On a personal level nurses, especially if they have had a recent bereavement, can find it difficult. One thing that might help nurses communicate in a more patient-centred, sensitive and supportive way in a situation that they find very stressful themselves is to realize that they are not there to make the person feel better. This is probably the worst day of that person's life so to think that as a nurse they can make it better is very presumptuous and sets an unachievable goal for the nurse. However a nurse can help the person in a number of different ways. These include:

- give the family as much time as they need – it can take a whole morning to help a family after ensuring that you have met their needs and given them all the information they require;
- bring the person or family to a private area;
- offer beverages; and
- stay with the family even if no one is talking. This does not mean that you are not needed. They may suddenly think of a question about how the person died or what happens next and if you are there to answer it will help them get through the day. It is always best not to talk too much, silence may be difficult for the nurse but can be comforting for the bereaved because they will be lost in their own thoughts. They will talk if they want to and all the nurse needs to do is listen. If as a nurse you have an intense need to talk it can result in you making a judgemental comment

or unconsciously agreeing when a family member blames himself or herself. For example:

> *Wife*: I last saw John (the dead person) when I brought him a cup of tea in the living room. He was watching TV and he said thanks when I put it down beside him. The phone rang then and it was Louise, our daughter and when I went back in to him, he wasn't breathing. That's when I called the ambulance.
> *Nurse*: How long were you on the phone for?
> *Wife*: About half an hour, perhaps if I had gone back in sooner??

Regardless of the reason for the nurse asking this question, it gave the wife feelings of guilt and added to her distress. The only time a nurse needs to talk is to answer questions asked and reassure the family and relatives in any way they can. Non-verbal communication is probably more effective in situations like this.

Bad news

Being present when a patient hears bad news can be upsetting for all involved. Sometimes the doctor and nurse will plan together how the patient will hear the news or the nurse may just be present when the doctor gives the patient the news, but usually after the patient hears the news and some explanation about what will happen next, the doctor leaves the room. The nurse should remain with the patient to support them, clarify information and answer any questions they might have. Key principles apply to any situation where a patient hears bad news:

- the nurse needs to ensure that they have time to spend with the patient. Do not appear hurried or rushed, as this will make the patient feel that they are keeping you from something more important. Spending time with the patient may be immediately after they hear the news or shortly afterwards. Sometimes the patient might want to be left alone or with family when they hear bad news but it is important that the nurse returns in a specified amount of time to talk to the patient;

- do not make assumptions about what information the patient wants. If you are unsure ASK THE PATIENT! 'Hi John, would you like to talk about what the doctor told you?;
- before giving any information ask the patient if they have any questions. This means that the information they receive is pertinent or important to them at that time. A number of visits may be required because the patient will need to have information repeated as people generally only retain 60 per cent of what they hear in normal situations and if they are very anxious they are likely to hear even less. They will also think of questions as they reflect on the news they received and try to make plans for the future when they are alone or discussing the news with their family;
- it is important to find out what the patient knows about their illness and the implications of the news they have heard. When this is established it is essential to determine what information the patient wants to hear. The only way to do this is to talk to the patient and ask them to tell you what they know. Follow their lead and observe their emotional behaviour as they do this. If a patient is not giving a great deal of information, by asking them directly if they would like more information on their illness, they will indicate very quickly how much information they want; and
- if they request more information ask them if they would like to have a family member present. This can be reassuring for them and two people can remember more than one.

Even though information concerning a patient is confidential, sometimes a doctor does not give the patient the bad news, instead the next of kin and family are informed first. The family may then decide to tell the patient themselves or ask the doctor to tell them. Although legally and ethically no one has the right to, occasionally the next of kin and family decide not to tell the patient the news because they feel that the patient would not want to hear the news. This is known as collusion and can create difficulties for nurses as they care for the patient as their physical condition deteriorates. The patient may ask the nurse why they are not getting better and because the nurse cannot explain what is happening to the patient, the patient can feel very confused and isolated. In order to prevent such scenarios the nurse can respond to a request not to tell the patient anything in a number of ways:

> *Family member:* Nurse the doctor has just told me and my family that John's cancer has spread and all they can offer is palliative care. We don't want John to know about this because it would only upset him and make him lose hope.
>
> *Nurse:* I understand that but as a nurse I think it is important to find out what John already knows or suspects about what is happening to him. He may not be saying anything because he is trying to protect all of you. Maybe I should talk to him and see if he knows anything and, if he does, maybe you should all get together and talk?
>
> *Family member:* And what if he doesn't seem to know anything?
>
> *Nurse:* In that case there may not be any need for you to talk at the moment, however, I should tell you that if he asks me anything about his illness, I cannot withhold information and will answer his questions truthfully.

Grief and bereavement

Death and dying is one particular area where students and newly qualified nurses find it difficult to use theory to inform their practice, and probably for good reason. Theory related to bereavement and grief is usually centred on the work of theorists such as Kubler-Ross (1973), Engel (1972) and Lindemann (1944). Lindemann's (1944) theory emphasizes the immediate physical reaction that people experience when they hear bad news or a relative/friend dies. This response includes tightness in the throat, shortness of breath, sighing, feeling empty and a lack of muscle power. Intense emotional distress accompanies the physical response. Engel's (1972) theory describes the bereavement process in stages. These include:

1. shock, disbelief, denial;
2. developing awareness;
3. re-institution phase;
4. resolving the loss; and
5. idealization phase.

Similarly Kubler-Ross's theory identifies five stages to the bereavement process. These include:

1. denial and isolation;
2. anger;
3. bargaining;
4. depression; and
5. acceptance

Although perhaps relevant to some people's experiences of bereavement, the work of Kubler-Ross (1973) and others who refer to dealing with bereavement as a series of stages is increasingly criticized by social scientists. The stages are useful in that they comprise descriptions of a variety of emotional responses to bad news and bereavement; the use of the term 'stages' indicates that an individual progresses through each stage either sequentially or at some point in their grieving/ bereavement process. Therefore, when a nurse witnesses a reaction that does not fit any of these descriptions, they can perceive it as abnormal. An example of this is when people from some cultures hear bad news or are bereaved they demonstrate their distress physically by throwing themselves on the floor or wailing. Other cultures, particularly Western cultures exhibit a more restrained response to grief and bereavement. The following quote is from a woman talking about the death of her 11 week old baby and demonstrates the typical response to grief and bereavement in the Western culture. 'I wanted to shout and scream – to tear my hair out – to keen. But I didn't. I behaved like a first-world woman and just cried until there was nothing left' (Anonymous, 1994).

It is important, therefore, as a nurse to respect any response that a person has to bad news or bereavement even if it is not the reaction that you personally would expect.

Grief and bereavement are different for individuals and the perception that a person needs to experience predetermined stages of grieving before they are regarded as 'over it' is perhaps not appropriate. For example, if a person cries when talking about a relative or friend that died one to two years previously, it may be perceived that they have not progressed through the bereavement stages and are having an abnormal bereavement reaction. Counselling is frequently seen as the solution to helping someone move on with their life and sometimes individuals may find it useful. However Craib (1999) believes that a different attitude towards grief and bereavement or death and dying can result in a very different approach to helping a person cope. 'Mourning never comes to an end; it is a process of remembering not one of leaving behind. The people we have lost live on within us and we can continue our relationship with them' (Craib, 1999, p. 89)

By accepting that grief and bereavement is a normal reaction that can vary enormously between individuals rather than a series of stages to go through, a nurse can help a person deal with bad news or the death of a relative or friend in a more person-centred way. This means that by just being with the person and not having any expectations about how they should behave, the nurse may feel less anxious about how a person will react. The reaction of the person is almost irrelevant to how a nurse can help an individual or family, it is the reaction of the nurse that determines whether he/she can be supportive and helpful in this very difficult situation. The following actions by the nurse are important:

● maintain a physical presence with the person or family – close physical presence or a discrete distance may be appropriate;
● actively listen and let silence happen – this allows the person or family to think; and
● provide verbal and written information about what happens to the body and what the family need to do.

Supporting a person or family that have just lost a relative or friend is very emotionally draining and tiring for a nurse. When the bereaved have left the ward, the nurse might find it psychologically and physically helpful to take a break before getting on with the rest of the day's work.

One of the comments made frequently by students in relation to communication classes on dealing with grief and bereavement is that even if the class content is relevant, it still doesn't teach them how to do this in reality. This could be because students do not know what is expected from them in these situations when really, as we have seen from the above discussion, all that is required is an empathetic presence and the provision of information at the appropriate time regarding what happens next for the family. Other possible reasons why students and qualified staff nurses find it difficult to communicate include:

- lack of confidence in relation to their own communication ability. Learning to be comfortable with silence and actively listen are the primary skills required when dealing with the dying and people who are bereaved; and
- dealing with death and dying at work on a regular basis can be a constant reminder of our own mortality and that of family and friends. Spending time thinking about how you feel about death and your own spirituality could help you feel less anxious when helping others that are bereaved and grieving. Answering the questions in the exercise below, either on your own or with friends, may help you identify your thoughts and feelings.

 Exercise

How do you feel when you think about your own death?
Would you like to be cremated or buried when you die?
How would you like to die?
Do you believe in life after death?

Trying to answer these questions may make you feel uneasy but it will allow you to clearly separate your own personal views on death and dying from those of the people you care for at work. It means that when you communicate with people who are dying you are less fearful of questions like 'Nurse am I dying?' Because although the situation is still difficult, you may now be more comfortable with the emotions that you feel in relation to the topic, having explored them. This will allow you to give a patient-centred response, for example, 'What makes you think that you are dying?'

Cross-cultural communication

In the previous section we mentioned how people from different cultures often react to grief and bereavement in a very specific way. In this section the difficulties that can exist with communication between people from different cultural backgrounds because of the meaning attributed to various aspects of verbal and non-verbal communication will be discussed. Most societies are now multicultural and while this is not generally an issue of concern for people in their personal lives, it has considerable implications for those working in health care provision. The ability to provide intercultural care is based on an inherent respect for other people and a knowledge and understanding of the concept of culture and its influence on the behaviour of patients and nurses and other health care workers from different countries, or those that represent different cultures within the same country.

Although often associated with race, the term 'ethnicity' actually refers to groups with a common cultural heritage and sense of identity. In contrast, the term 'race' is associated with biology, with members of a particular race sharing features such as skin colour (Giger and Davidhizar, 1999). Ethnic and racial groups often overlap because of the biological and cultural similarities they share. Many definitions of culture exist but most share the common belief that culture represents the values, beliefs, norms and practices of a particular group that are learned, shared and guide thinking, decisions and actions in a specific way (Giger and Davidhizar, 1999).

Factors within ethnic groups, such as gender, age, education, religion, and socio-economic status result in cultural diversity within an ethnic group. This means that for nurses to care for patients with different cultural backgrounds in a patient-centred way they need to determine what aspects of a patient's culture are significant to their care and how this influences the way the nurse needs to communicate on an individual basis. Leininger (1991) refers to this process as 'transcultural nursing' and suggests that nurses need knowledge about many cultural values, beliefs and practices in order to provide individual and holistic nursing care. Nurses and midwives, however, do not always communicate well with patients with different cultural and religious backgrounds (Jones and Van Amelsvoort-Jones, 1986; Stockwell, 1972; Windsor-Richards and Gillies, 1988; Wollett and Dosanjh-Matwala, 1990). This can be because if a nurse does not understand the patient's language they may avoid trying to communicate with the patient because it is embarrassing or time consuming. Waiting for the family to come in is a more efficient option. However, in the meantime the patient may be feeling isolated, uncomfortable and frightened. Often words are not necessary for a nurse to provide comfort and support when waiting for family or an interpreter to translate. Smiling or using gestures and gentle touch can be a very effective communication approach when trying to comfort and support a patient.

Some cultures are very expressive and use their hands, facial expression and voices to communicate in a way that can be perceived as argumentative or loud. This behaviour may also be perceived as unnecessary and aggressive by less expressive cultures. A nurse may regard such behaviour as demanding or even intimidating and may avoid the patient or be defensive. The list of differences and similarities between cultures and ethnic groups is long, and perhaps in terms of how a nurse communicates in a patient-centred way, is irrelevant. We support Lea's (1994) view that for transcultural communication to be successful, nurses need to be aware of their own cultural values and attitudes and how these influence their perceptions of patients and the nursing care they give. This may sound familiar to you because we discussed the importance of developing awareness of how you communicate in order to be patient-centred in Chapters 3 and 9. The same principal applies for transcultural communication and helps prevent assumptions being made about a person's behaviour. In other words, the nurse can give a rational and non-judgemental response to patients regardless of their cultural or ethnic background.

Ethnocentrism may be a problem for nurses who are not aware of their own cultural values and attitudes. 'This is the perception that one's own way is best' (Giger and Davidhizar, 1999, p. 66). They suggest that nurses have a tendency towards ethnocentrism and this is evident in the way nurses often make assumptions about what patients need and provide nursing care without asking the patient what they want. For example, Western culture views health and illness as a biophysical process and this is reflected in nurses' tendency to deal with the physical needs of a patient as separate from their psychological needs and well-being whereas other cultures, such as some Puerto Ricans, believe that illness is related to evil or many Ugandans relate illness with being cursed (Grypma, 1993). Awareness of oneself as an unique individual with a cultural and ethnic background allows a nurse to view others also as unique individuals with individual needs and provide patient-centred care. Methods of developing self-awareness will be further developed in Chapter 9.

Key points

▶ Situations are sometimes perceived as 'difficult' by nurses because of a perceived lack of communication skills.

▶ Ordinary everyday situations can become 'difficult' because nurses communicate inappropriately or negatively.

▶ Observing a 'good' role model is a very effective way of developing effective and positive communication skills.

▶ The key to managing 'difficult' situations is to learn to 'manage yourself'. This requires self-awareness, motivation and practice.

▶ A key role of the nurse in situations relating to death/dying, bereavement and bad news is to provide comfort and information that is helpful, relevant and patient-centred.

▶ Learning to managing anxiety (nurse's and patient's) will alleviate or possibly prevent, many 'difficult' situations.

▶ Awareness of personal cultural values and attitudes is essential in preventing ethnocentrism and allows nurses to care for patients from other cultures in a patient-centred and individualized way.

7 Resolving conflict

Introduction

In this chapter assertive behaviour and negotiation skills are viewed as essential skills in allowing nurses to be autonomous practitioners within a multidisciplinary team. Assertive behaviour is described as a person giving expression to his/her rights, thoughts and feelings without denying the rights of others (Alberti and Emmons, 1986). These skills are also considered integral to allowing nurses to communicate within the multidisciplinary team as an advocate for patients, and working collaboratively within the multidisciplinary team in caring for patients.

Overview of conflict

Conflict is regarded as a natural part of the clinical environment within which many nurses and nursing students operate (Balzer-Riley, 2000; Gregory Dawes, 1999; Underman Boggs, 2003). Taylor (1989) suggested that conflict is an inevitable part of life and that it is not preventing conflict that is important but helping people to manage themselves and the situations they are in more successfully. How conflict is handled is one sign of the health and effectiveness of the group's functioning. Healthy, open conflict can promote individual commitment and participation in the activity in which they are taking part (Taylor, 1989). Alternatively, conflict that is stifled or brought to a premature close can delay progress, limit discussion of the range of options and lead to accumulation of resentment that can resurface at a later date (Taylor, 1989).

Gregory Dawes (1999) suggested that conflict:

is a human influencing option that is neither positive nor negative until we direct the energy patterns that are generated from conflict. As conflict often involves explosive emotions, people are intimidated by the situation. Like unresolved stress, conflict results in low productivity and promotes mediocre performance, boredom, and apathy. In turn, it creates more stress.

Gregory Dawes (1999) also suggested that conflict arises from a perception of incompatibility. It emanates from differences in beliefs, values, goals, priorities, methods, information, commitments, ideas, and interpretations of reality, backgrounds, needs, interests and/or motives. It is a manifestation of unclear expectations, poor communication, lack of clear jurisdiction, disagreements based on different attitudes/ temperaments, and individual or group conflicts of interest. Within nursing it can also emanate from operational and staffing shortages (Gregory Dawes, 1999). Causes of conflict as outlined by Underman Boggs (2003) include poor communication, differences in values and goals, personality clashes and stress. Underman Boggs (2003) also suggested that conflict between nurse and patient is not uncommon.

Definition of conflict

But what precisely is meant by conflict? Taylor (1989, p. 60) identifies conflict as 'the more an individual defines the situation as one in which they can only gain their goal at the expense of others, the more conflict is likely.' Taylor also suggested that three principal types of conflict exist: controversies, conflicts over needs and developmental conflicts. Conflict arises once incompatible activities occur in a pair, a group or an organization. Incompatible activities confront those involved with questions of priority and, therefore, issues of choice. It involves feelings because 'emotions are an inevitable accompaniment to what people want – people care about what they do and how they do it, whether it will be done now or later, and who will be involved in doing it with them' (Taylor, 1989, p. 60). If conflict and differences are genuine they will not go away by simply pushing them aside, although this is a common method of attempting to resolve conflict.

Although people can be uncomfortable with conflict, Taylor (1989, p. 61) suggested that conflict itself is 'rarely destructive or damaging'. It is, rather, its inadequate management that brings about the distress, the violence, the disorder and the disintegration which occurs around it. Groups may benefit from conflict as apathy can occur in organizations where it is stifled. 'Open, healthy challenge in our organizational life is relatively rare.' Benefits of conflict as expressed by Taylor include an increase in the awareness of the complexity of issues, an encouragement to change and respond in an active way and increased decision making. It may also increase individual awareness, reduce tension, and promote feelings of engagement either to the group, the task, or both.

Underman Boggs (2003) defined conflict as tension arising from incompatible needs. Taylor (1989, p. 62) found that conflicts over needs and values are often characterized not by open exchanges but by 'a stifling of the differences which attempts to overlook the real issues of choice and priority that are contained within the conflict itself.' Assignment of priorities, the allocation of resources, decisions that have implications for members of staff, client groups, friends and neighbours are areas where conflict is avoided in the hope of an alternative solution, which rarely occurs. These can, therefore, carry an accumulation of distress much more than if the issues were dealt with at an early stage.

Developmental conflicts have within them the potential for movement and change. Often they represent conflicts about issues such as relocation, readjustment, response to new demands, and to changes in activities and purposes. They are primarily the kinds of conflict that we find in the work place although they can occur in families during readjustment periods. Organizational changes and relocation of departments are other examples.

There are six major elements to consider for constructive use of conflict: the definition of the problem; levels and accuracy of information; the climate in which the disputes are being managed; the value of the activity over which the conflict is taking place; the response to and respect for the feelings of those involved; and a recognition of similarities as well as differences on behalf of those taking part (Taylor, 1989).

While agreeing that conflict is a natural part of human interactions Balzer-Riley (2000, p. 372) suggested that 'it can have advantageous outcomes when it is handled in assertive and responsible ways'. They suggested that conflict arises when interdependency exists. Conflicts can occur about facts, methods, goals and values. Conflict can occur within an individual (intrapersonal), between individuals (interpersonal) within a group (intragroup) or between groups (intergroup) (Balzer-Riley, 2000). Resolution of conflict in the workplace situation means acting in such a way that agreement is reached that is acceptable and pleasing to all parties. Balzer-Riley (2000) also suggested assertiveness as a response to overcome conflict. Taylor (1989) also supported the use of assertiveness skills to deal with conflict.

Common responses to conflict

Four styles commonly used in response to conflict are avoidance, accommodation, competition and collaboration (Underman Boggs, 2003). The latter is a solution-orientated approach whereby a mutually satisfactory solution is reached. Gender differences to conflict management have been suggested and Valentine (1995, 2001) found that women predominately used the conflict management strategies of avoiding and compromising. Underman Boggs (2003) also suggested that the nature of the nursing profession might promote conflict avoidance. 'Nurses traditionally were socialized to follow orders. Women were socialized not to 'make waves" (Underman Boggs, 2003, p. 369).

Baker (1995) and Aschenbrener and Siders (1999) identified five behavioural actions that are usually taken by individuals during conflict:

1. Competing;
2. Compromising;
3. Avoiding;
4. Accommodating; and
5. Collaborating.

Competing is usually characterized by aggressive or uncooperative behaviour. *Compromising* may result in a quick closure, but decisions may be made in haste. *Avoidance* involves ignoring the situation and not addressing the issue. Gregory Dawes (1999) identified several research studies of conflict resolution that provided evidence that nurses overuse avoidance as a conflict resolution method. *Accommodating* behaviour is a cooperative approach, but it reinforces unassertive behaviour and may foster apathy in the workplace (Gregory Dawes, 1999).

Collaborating directly addresses the issue or conflict. It is characterized by problem identification and open dialogue that leads to mutually satisfactory conclusions. Collaboration promotes effective communication and problem solving, because both individuals try to seek mutually agreeable solutions (Baker, 1995; McElhaney, 1996). Both parties set aside their original goals and work together to establish a supraordinate or common goal. The focus in collaboration is problem solving, rather than defeating the other party.

Gregory Dawes (1999) suggested that although these behaviours (avoidance, accommodating and compromise) are used regularly and may have a place in everyday interactions, a collaborative approach to conflict resolution is the most appropriate, because it involves using problem-solving skills, cooperation and open communication, all of which are important social skills for the health care professional.

Dealing with conflict

An estimated 20 per cent of managerial time is spent dealing with conflict (Valentine, 2001). When conflict is handled inappropriately, demoralization, decreased motivation and lower productivity commonly occur (Gregory Dawes, 1999). Conflict resolution requires separating information in a conflict situation, consideration of what factors contribute to the conflict, and actual problem-solving techniques. Problem-solving techniques include identifying the problem, brainstorming solutions, and asking if the solution is safe, fair, and how others will feel about it. After implementing the solution, ongoing evaluation is always necessary to monitor the conflict and make amends as needed.

Taylor (1989, p. 72) described costs and benefits to actions within conflict situations, suggesting, 'if you always do what you always did, you will always get what you always got'. He suggested that using assertiveness in situations can assist people to do things differently and become more effective in not only resolving conflict but also in improving their own well-being. It is important, Taylor (1989) pointed out, to try out new assertiveness skills in manageable situations as taking on too much too soon can lead to disappointment:

> In work places where the resolution of conflict is avoided, where disputes are displaced, where differences are discounted, the active use of assertiveness skills in the short term may create more difficulties for the person concerned than by continuing to go along with the culture of the group or the work place itself. Those who are considering implementing assertiveness skills need to pay careful attention to the culture of the organization, work group or team in which they intend to act, and the likely consequences in the short and long term of implementing such behaviors. (Taylor 1989).

Underman Boggs (2003) clearly suggested that conflict could serve either a functional or dysfunctional role in relationships. They clearly outlined assertive behaviour as the main course of action for conflict situations. They suggested that this involves 'setting goals, acting on those goals in a clear and consistent manner, and taking responsibility for the consequences of those actions. The assertive nurse is able to stand up for the rights of others as well as his or her own rights' (2003, p. 373). They outlined principles of conflict resolution: identify conflict issues, know your own response to conflict, separate the problem from the people involved, stay focused on the issue and on the underlying motivations behind the position the other person took, identify available options, try to identify established standards to guide the decision-making process.

When applying this to the nurse–patient relationship Underman Boggs (2003) suggested assessing the presence of conflict in the nurse–patient relationship by using nursing strategies to enhance conflict resolution. Underman Boggs (2003, p. 381) outlined several strategies for dealing with interpersonal conflict. These included developing assertive skills; demonstrating respect for others; using 'I' statements (rather than 'you'); making statements that are clear, using appropriate pitch and tone; being able to analyse personal feelings in the situation and focus on the present. They also describe how to deal with encounters in nursing practice with angry patients or relatives. They suggest using communication skills to look for early non-verbal clues; once identified, the feeling could be labelled. For example you could say 'You seem angry?'

They also suggest that you may give permission for anger within limits. This may be demonstrated by the statement 'it is perfectly understandable that you are angry in this situation.' This also helps the person to own the anger feelings. Acknowledging the person's feelings is an important first step in the resolution process. Rather than the nurse talking excessively or trying to use words to resolve the situation, using communication skills identified earlier in the book, a series of open questions and attentive listening may elicit why the person is angry. This may be very productive in diffusing the situation. By then identifying what it is that has triggered the anger, the nurse may be able to assist the person to develop a simple plan to deal with the situation. Thus active listening, a key component of the therapeutic relationship, prevents the escalation of conflict (Arnold, 2003).

Other therapeutic listening responses can also be useful in this situation, such as using minimal cues and avoiding leading questions. Thus rather than saying 'you are annoyed because your visitors had to leave early' you would elicit more information and be less likely to aggravate the situation by using the statement 'tell me what is going on for you right now.' In a conflict situation with a patient or visitor, it is important to use the self-awareness that you have developed to prevent yourself from jumping in and providing a range of responses to the situation. Once a response has been elicited from the open question, it can be clarified 'so you're telling me that you are cross because visiting time seemed to be very short today', summarized or paraphrased. Silence can also be used if appropriate. The nurse's response must be calm with use of appropriate vocabulary, with a view to focusing the situation to the problem and presenting reality. In this case, the visiting times may be unavoidable, and this could be explained, however, providing empathy in a situation of disappointment might serve to ease the tension. Similarly, there may be room for an apology if the visitor was rushed away in a manner that wasn't appropriate.

Arnold (2003) also suggested using humour, which she describes as 'a powerful communication technique when it is used with deliberate intent for a specific therapeutic purpose' (Arnold, 2003, p. 257). Humour would obviously need to be used appropriately, but can be used to show one's authentic self and can diffuse tension in some situations.

Using assertive skills

Taylor (1989) and Underman Boggs (2003) suggested using assertiveness as a method of dealing with conflict. Although commonly thought to be personality trait, assertiveness is a form of behaviour that can be learned (Rakos, 2003; Willis and Daisley, 1995). It is also situation specific; thereby its use can be selective (Rakos, 2003). It involves specific responses, seven of which were described in a review by Schroeder *et al.* in 1983. These included four positive responses: admitting shortcomings (self-disclosure); giving and receiving compliments; initiating and maintaining interactions; and expressing positive feelings. Three negative or conflict responses included expressing unpopular or different opinions; requesting behaviour changes by others; and refusing unreasonable requests.

Rakos (2003) suggested that a plethora of research in the area of assertive behaviour has taken place over the past 25 years. Rakos suggested that assertion rose to prominence as a social skill in the mid 1970s as a pop psychology fad and as a clinical focus of behaviour therapy. Assertion and assertive behaviour are also gaining increasing popularity within the nursing literature as evidenced by the title of the opening chapter in Balzer Riley (2000, p. xv) 'Responsive, Assertive, Caring Communication in Nursing'. Clearly for this author assertive behaviour is central to the nursing role and is interdependent with the caring behaviours required of the nurse.

However, there are barriers in the workplace that prevent the use of assertive skills by nurses. Poroch and McIntosh (1995) identified some of these barriers. These included a lack of knowledge about personal/professional rights; concern about what others will think about their behaviour; and anxiety due to a lack of confidence and poor self-esteem. This overriding concern with how others (the public and other health professionals) view assertive behaviour among nurses permeates throughout the literature.

Rakos (2003) suggested that individual perceptions and beliefs could predict assertive behaviour. Those less likely to behave assertively are more likely to have a need for perfection in themselves and others, and be inclined towards blaming themselves and/or others for imperfect behaviour. They also require universal and unwavering approval from others and may define self-worth by external achievement. These individuals would also view passive behaviour as the preferable option, safe in the belief that 'things will work out eventually'.

Balzer-Riley (2000, p. 8) defined assertive communication in the nursing context as 'the key to successful relationships for the client, family, the nurse, and other colleagues. It is the ability to express your thoughts, your ideas, and your feelings without undue anxiety and without expense to others'. She suggested, 'the assertive nurse appears confident and comfortable.' She also pointed out that assertive communication is a skill that may be learned over a lifetime and it is also a matter of choice.

She also noted that it might be difficult to make choices about assertive behaviour during situations where a person is 'experiencing high levels of anxiety or panic' (Balzer-Riley, 2000, p. 10). This is important to recognize within the health care setting. Patients and families are often experiencing these feelings and, therefore, an expectation that these persons would communicate assertively is unrealistic. While verbal and physical abuse is clearly intolerable in these settings, it is up to the nurse not to react inappropriately where consumers present with aggressive, passive, manipulative or defensive behaviour. The nurse is in a better position, due to their lack of direct attachment and emotional involvement with recipients of care, to reflect maturely and consider the situation and choose an appropriate response should these behaviours occur. A relative, for example, who approaches the nurse while he/she is sitting writing reports at his/her desk, stands closely above the nurse, points their finger and shouts 'my mother has not been to the toilet all morning'. An assertive response would include asking the relative to sit down, or standing to assume the same height. Then reflecting back the question 'your mother has not been to the toilet all morning, tell me a little more about that'. Allowing the person to express their feelings in this regard, would allow some of the pent up aggression to abate. By maintaining eye contact, speaking in a quiet/normal voice in conjunction with the previous sentence the nurse encourages a more assertive response. In this case the reason for the outburst related to the relative's upset and feeling of powerlessness at their mother's declining memory. She had actually been to the toilet frequently that morning and the nurse was able to demonstrate this using the nursing notes. The relative's frustration that had been redirected at the nursing staff emerged from an emotional reaction to the mothers' illness. Once assertiveness skills were used, open person-centred communication allowed the relative to share many of these feelings. Assertiveness is often discussed synonymously with 'rights'. Commonly known as assertive rights an example of this is provided in Figure 7.1.

Although not implicit in this Figure, assertiveness is also based on the premise that the other person within the inter-action also has equal rights. From the earlier example, the nurse in the previous scenario could have expressed his/her feelings thus: 'I feel very embarrassed that this may have occurred, let me investigate this further for you.' One of the key aspects of assertive behaviour is that, while exerting rights may be an expression of personal beliefs and opinions, it does not actually confer those rights. For example, the right for you to make mistakes cannot be imposed on others. You cannot insist that others give you the right to make mistakes. What knowing and understanding your rights does is confer upon you an understanding of, and confidence in, your basic human rights that you may use to assist your self-awareness and assertiveness in a given situation. However, attaining those rights is not the goal of the assertive communication but

- I have the right to express my own feelings and opinions
- I have the right to state my own needs and set my own priorities as a person, independent of any roles that I may assume in life
- I have the right to be treated with respect as an intelligent, capable and equal human being
- I have the right to say 'no' or 'yes' for myself
- I have the right to make mistakes – and be responsible for them
- I have the right to change my mind
- I have the right to say 'I don't understand' and to ask for more information
- I have the right to ask for what I want
- I have the right to decline responsibility for other peoples problems
- I have the right to deal with people without being dependent on them for approval

Source: McCabe, C. and Timmins, F. (2003) Teaching assertiveness to undergraduate nursing students *Nurse Education in Practice*, 3(1), 30–42, with permission from Elsevier.

Figure 7.1 Assertive rights

rather the expression of them. Bearing in mind however, as Taylor (1989) pointed out; assertive behaviour may not be appropriate in all situations. Taylor (1989) also suggested that when assertive behaviour is relatively new to a person, it may be best to try out new techniques in a relatively safe environment, for example when returning an item to a shop, rather than reserving first attempts for contentious issues or conflict situations, where skills require more practice.

Assertiveness is an interpersonal behaviour that is defined as:

> that which attends to and informs others of one's own needs and feelings and sends the message to the other in such a way that neither person is belittled, put down or blamed. (Poritt, 1990, p. 98)

Assertive behaviour is also described as a person giving expression to his/her rights, thoughts and feelings without denying the rights of others (Alberti and Emmons, 1986). Taylor (1989) suggested that within conflict, one of the most common situations to involve assertiveness skills, perceptions of the situation by the parties involved are quite different. Negotiating understandings is important. Taylor (1989) suggested that the benefits of using assertiveness in the management of conflict are: improved relationships; improving trust and openness; increase in satisfaction; and improvement in decision making. Taylor (1989, p. 5) suggested that assertion was 'about making oneself visible to others, standing up for oneself, if you like, in a way that seeks recognition and acknowledgement rather than insists upon being given in to'. Taylor further distinguishes the 'assertive response' as combining the four C's: clarity of communication; congruence of response; consistency about the issue; and collaboration – inviting the other person to engage in this issue. Congruence is the 'match between what you say and what you do, what you say and how you feel', incongruence, he suggested, as described in Chapter 1, may be picked up by others and may reduce the impact of your attempts at assertiveness. Clarity involves stating a point simply, identifying the issues and sticking to it. It may mean repeating the point again and again. When an individual is not behaving assertively, responses can be categorized as aggressive, passive, manipulative or defensive.

Aggressive responses

Aggressive responses involve an attempt to use personal anger to persuade the other person. This can involve body language such as proximity (standing too close to another) or finger wagging. Taylor (1989) suggested that this should not be confused with anger. Expressing anger can be useful in a situation, and may be done assertively, for example saying in a normal voice tone: 'I feel angry that I have to work next Sunday, I had made prior arrangements.' However, in this situation the person is simply expressing their feelings openly without expecting the other to act upon it. When aggression is used there is a deliberate attempt to persuade or punish the other individual in the interaction. The use of a loud voice, and aggressive body language (finger wagging, standing over the other) all contribute to the aggressive message. Passive responses on the other hand are aimed at quiet manipulation. This could include withdrawal, for example refusing to contribute within a team meeting or quietly refusing to implement new ways of working. The defensive response according to Taylor (1989) occurs where individuals have a sense of belonging over something (for example territory, equipment or regulations). At the slightest imposition the person rises to defend, without considering the other's viewpoint and it can quickly escalate into aggression. Willis and Daisley (1995) described aggression as seeking to get your own way regardless of the consequences. This can be indirect and not that obvious or loud; or violent and abusive with interruptions and intimidation. The results of aggression are arguments that are won at the expense of others, causing people to be annoyed and the aggressor to be disliked and freaked.

The manipulative response

The manipulative response Taylor (1989) suggested is one of the most common responses to conflict, particularly in situations and cultures where open conflict or direct confrontation are discouraged. Those using manipulation try to take the focus away from the person who is trying to express an opinion. By changing the topic, minimizing or scoffing at the suggestion the subject is inevitably changed. This behaviour 'frustrate[s] the efforts of others into giving up on an issue' (Taylor, 1989, p. 26).

The passive response

Passive behaviour, Willis and Daisley (1995, p. 10) suggested, is keeping quiet so as not to upset others; keeping thoughts and feelings internalized; 'saying yes when you want to say no'; excessive apologizing; and appearing indecisive while actually knowing what one wants. The results of passive behaviour is that arguments are lost, the person may be considered a *doormat* or a victim, the person remains indeci-

Assertive behaviour:

- Being open and honest with yourself and other people
- Listening to other people's point of view
- Showing an understanding of other people's situations
- Expressing your ideas clearly, but not at the expense of others
- Being able to reach workable solutions to difficulties
- Making decisions – even if your decision is not to make a decision!
- Being clear about your point and not being sidetracked
- Dealing with conflict
- Speaking up
- Having self-respect and respect for other people
- Being equal with others while restating your uniqueness
- Expressing your feelings honestly but with care
- Standing up for yourself

Results of assertive behaviour:

- Conflicts are resolved openly
- Potential difficult situations are dealt with early
- Confidence increases
- Fear reduces as skills are developed in handling emotional situations
- People become equal with others while retaining their uniqueness
- There Is recognition of the effect of behaviour on others
- People retain their dignity

Source: adapted from Willis, L. and Daisley, J. (1995) *The Assertive Trainer: A Practical Handbook for Trainers and Running Assertiveness Courses,* Maidenhead: McGraw-Hill Book Company Europe.

Figure 7.2 Assertive behaviour and results

sive and may become 'bitter later in life' (Willis and Daisley, 1995, p. 11). The overriding motto of passive behaviour is 'anything for a quiet life' (Willis and Daisley, 1995, p. 11). Assertive behaviour on the other hand is quite different (Willis and Daisley, 1995) and is displayed in Figure 7.2.

The assertive response

Willis and Daisley (1995, p. 12) described assertive behaviour thus: 'assertiveness is a form of behaviour which demonstrates

> - Listen
> - Demonstrate that you understand the other person
> - Say what you think and feel
> - Say specifically what you want to happen
> - Consider the consequences for yourself and others of any joint solutions

Source: adapted from Willis, L. and Daisley, J. (1995) *The Assertive Trainer: A Practical Handbook for Trainers and Running Assertiveness Courses*, Maidenhead: McGraw-Hill Book Company Europe.

Figure 7.3 Five vital components of assertiveness

your self-respect and respect for others. This means that assertiveness is concerned with dealing with your own feelings about yourself and other people, as much as with the end result.' There are five vital ingredients according to Willis and Daisley (1995) (Figure 7.3)

They also focused upon 'getting assertive words' (Willis and Daisley, 1995, p. 24), suggesting that having an understanding of what assertiveness is doesn't necessarily mean that personal behaviours will follow. It is important to speak in a way that is open, clear, constructive and in a voice that is steady, firm, warm, clear, sincere, neither loud nor soft and audible. A voice that is fast, pompous, loud, strident, sharp, abrupt, shouting, clipped or sarcastic, and that uses excessive emphasis on words, threatening statements or criticism, conveys aggression. Whereas being longwinded, apologetic, self-critical, soft, hesitant, tentative, slow/quiet or fast/garbled can appear passive. They highlighted that the words that are spoken, 'your assertive script' (Willis and Daisley, 1995, p. 24), are only 7 per cent of the total message. They suggested (1995, p. 24) that to be assertive not only involves using assertive language but one must '*sound* assertive and *look* assertive whilst delivering them' (emphasis authors' own). This is an important aspect of learning and practising assertive behaviour skills (McCabe and Timmins, 2003).

Assertiveness 'typically has been conceptualized as the mid-point on the continuum between non-assertive (passive) and aggressive behaviour' (Rakos, 2003, p. 291). Other important components of assertiveness include paralinguistics, non-verbal behaviours and social interaction skills (timing, initiation, persistence) (Rakos, 2003).

Are nurses assertive?

Registered nurses adhere to rigorous guidelines and codes and are called to account for actions. Contemporary nursing is set in a context of evidence-based practice. As an accountable profession, nursing is continuously expanding its knowledge base through research and further education to maintain competence. Professional development (Brechin, 2000) is the cornerstone of modern nursing. Nursing roles are expanding to increase specialist knowledge and skills. The need for continued education for registration requirements and the increasing repertoire of evidence-based nursing interventions both indicate a highly organized professional group. However, there are factors extrinsic to nursing that influence not only their perceived professional status but may also cause conflict. Their position within the hospital health care team can positively or negatively affect these perceptions.

Nurses, although they are not the source of the primary diagnosis (Saks, 2000) and do not necessarily prescribe care, are by virtue of their regulation and position within the health care structure accountable for the care they provide. They are held to account for care often directed by others.

Nurses have extensive social, legal, ethical and professional accountability (Brechin, 2000). All of these aspects of accountability are quite separate in their definition; but form complex interplay that informs nurses' day to day practice. There is also extensive legal accountability that recognizes nurses' authority and liability in practice. This responsibility is pervasive, and not straightforward. Carrying out the orders of other professional groups has inherent liability for nurses involved. The latter can result in ethical dilemmas and conflicts, not always experienced by professional groups with greater autonomy. Underman Boggs (2003) suggested that it is these ethical dilemmas that cause an amount of conflict for nurses. In Dowling *et al.*'s (2000) case study for example, nurses refused to deliver inappropriate orders. The doctors opposed their views. The nurses had to embark on a formal procedure route to raise their concerns, which were upheld. These situations are not uncommon for nurses who often risk isolation and retaliation in the name of accountably, who may ultimately become 'whistleblowers', risking job loss, if not supported in the practice setting (Brechin, 2000).

McCartan (2001) reported a 'moderate' tendency for nurses to use assertion skills. However, assertive behaviour by nurses can be viewed as uncaring (Valentine, 1995). Percival (2001) suggested that nurses have to live up to their public image as 'nice' people, which militates against the use of assertive behaviour. Nice people usually accommodate and facilitate others, rather than asserting their own rights (Percival, 2001).

Poroch and McIntosh (1995) state that nurses feared rejection and isolation by colleagues if they used assertive, uncaring behaviour. The highest-ranking barrier to assertive behaviour in this group of nurses was the belief that it was uncaring behaviour. Timmins and McCabe (2005) noted that few nurses in their study had received assertiveness education and many respondents cited lack of knowledge as a barrier to using skills.

Furthermore, managers emerged as a main barrier to using assertive skills in this study (Timmins and McCabe, 2005). In addition, respondents used negative assertive skills less frequently with their mangers, although they often used positive skills (complementing and allowing them to voice opinions) (Timmins and McCabe, 2005). The workplace atmosphere either served as a barrier or facilitated assertive behaviour.

Assertive behaviour may conflict with the expectations of behaviour of a nice caring nurse (Farrell, 2001; Valentine, 1995; Percival, 2001). An interesting finding from Timmins and McCabe's (2005) study was that respondents (unprompted) cited responsibility to the patient as a primary facilitator of their assertive behaviour. Clearly, from these practicing clinicians' perspective, assertiveness is a requirement of patient care. This corresponds with the increasingly common role of nurses as a patient advocate as described by Domon

(1997). This is also congruent with Balzer-Riley's (2000) suggestion that assertiveness is a fundamental component of communication within the nurse–patient interaction and also of the therapeutic nurse–patient relationship. In her opening lines of the text 'Communication in Nursing' (Balzer-Riley, 2000) she suggested that the book was designed to help improve the 'ability to communicate assertively and responsibly with . . . clients and colleagues and demonstrate . . . caring'. Thus suggesting that assertiveness, communication and caring were fundamental and interlinked components of nursing practice. Indeed, a third of the book is devoted to the topic of assertiveness. This emphasis on assertiveness is both novel and unique within the nursing literature. In some texts a chapter may be devoted to the topic, in others it is not discussed. Given the deficits in assertive behaviour by nurses (Timmins and McCabe, 2005), together with the suggestion by nurses that their assertive behaviour was as a direct response to patient advocacy, we support Balzer-Riley's (2000) notion of the importance and centrality of assertiveness within the therapeutic nurse–patient relationship.

Consider the nurse working in Accident and Emergency, where people typically wait for up to four hours to be reviewed by a doctor. When passing by the long queue she is approached by a person who is not happy waiting in the queue. Adopting a defensive response 'we have a very busy department, you know, and if more people attended their GP it wouldn't be half as bad' may spark aggression in the person or simply cause hurt and embarrassment. Whereas an assertive approach 'I understand how frustrating that must be for you, is there anything I can do to help?', not only reduces the risk of bad feelings and reactions from the person waiting, but also allows open communication to begin, that is not focused on the nurse's problems but rather patient/person-centred.

It may well be that providing change for the telephone, or other simple solutions may ease the person's suffering in this case. Indeed clear information about the waiting times may also be useful, rather than a waiting time that is indefinite.

Patient-centred communication requires a continuing awareness by nurses as individuals of their contribution to interactions that they have not just with patients but also with relatives, friends, other health care professionals and health care staff. Therefore, the use by nurses of behaviours other than assertive behaviour with these consumers of health care limits the chance of the communication being truly patient-centred.

Key points

▶ Assertive behaviour and negotiation skills are regarded as essential skills, allowing nurses to be autonomous practitioners within a multi-disciplinary team.

▶ Conflict is inevitable in an environment where many healthcare disciplines work together. It can be positive but if it is not managed appropriately it can become negative and destructive.

▶ Collaboration is the most effective response to assertiveness because it facilitates the development of mutually satisfying solutions.

▶ Hierarchical health care structures and workplace atmospheres often are not only a cause of conflict but also prevent conflict from being managed successfully and positively.

PART III

The development of therapeutic communication skills

8 Values and beliefs in nursing

Introduction

The purpose of this chapter is to explore the values, beliefs and attitudes inherent in the nursing profession and how these influence the practice and development of nursing. This will be done in the context of nursing as a profession and how this guides and directs nursing. Students will find this chapter useful because it provides an explanation about what makes the work of a nurse unique within health care professions and how the values and beliefs that nurses hold about nursing are evident in how they communicate with patients, families and work colleagues. Concepts such as personal and professional values, ethics in nursing, professionalism and accountability will be discussed under separate headings in this chapter. However it is important to note that these concepts are inextricably linked in how they influence the practice and development of nursing.

Values

Values are made up of the beliefs and attitudes a person holds about everything in life. The values a person holds gives them meaning in what they do, how they appreciate their environment and people and guide how they react to situations in life (Tschudin, 2003). Values change and develop as we experience various aspects of life and often we are not aware of our values until they are tested, for example, a nurse may discover that although he/she does not agree with a patient refusing to undergo chemotherapy for the treatment of cancer, they value human rights and the patient's right to choose their treatment. The nurse, therefore, accepts the patient's decision and cares for them in this context.

Beliefs are influenced and guided by values; for example, a nurse may hold the value that every human being is an unique individual. In nursing this value will translate into the belief that maintaining the dignity and respect of the patient is the primary function of the nurse and should be reflected in the care that is given by the nurse.

An attitude is evident in a person's disposition and is formed by their values and beliefs. This can have a positive or negative influence on how a person communicates. Most of us recognize a positive or negative attitude in the way a person communicates verbally and non-verbally. In nursing, the belief that patients should do as they are told because the doctor or nurse knows best will translate into an attitude whereby the nurse does not respect the right of the individual to choose their treatment or even be involved in decisions about their treatment. This nurse may argue with the patient, try to coerce them and generally disregard the patient's viewpoint. This type of communication is not patient-centred and the patient may even be labelled as 'difficult'. The attitude or disposition of a nurse is influenced by their upbringing and environment but also, and probably most importantly, the values and beliefs they hold about human beings and the role of the nurse.

 Exercise

What values do you hold about nursing and your role as a nurse? If you are not sure, ask yourself the following questions:

Why did I choose nursing as a career?
What aspects of my job do I like the most?
What aspects of my job do I like the least?

Be honest with yourself when considering the answers to these questions, otherwise the exercise will not help you identify your real values about nursing and the role of the nurse. Knowing what you value about your job will give meaning to the job you do and may even boost your self-esteem. However, consider the answers carefully because as you read on in this chapter, you will see how your values impact greatly on how you do your job!

Defining nursing is generally regarded as problematic but according to this well-known quote from Virginia Henderson (1966):

> The unique function of the nurse is to assist the individual, sick or well, in the performance of those activities contributing to health or its recovery (or to a peaceful death) that he would perform unaided if he had the necessary strength, will or knowledge. And to do this in such a way as to help him gain independence as rapidly as possible.

This is a useful definition in providing a broad view of what nursing aspires to but further consideration suggests that this definition could also apply to other health care disciplines such as physiotherapists, occupational therapists and doctors. Also, what is lacking in this definition is the recognition of the integral contribution that the values, beliefs and attitudes of individual nurses make to the implementation of this role. In other words, how the nurse communicates this role to her patient. In earlier chapters we discussed Rogers' (1961) person-centred theory and how the personal characteristics of warmth, genuineness and unconditional positive regard are required to be person-centred. These characteristics go hand-in-hand with the personal values that regard human beings as unique individuals that deserve to be treated with respect and dignity. A person-centred attitude or approach to patient care will be evident in nurses with these values and characteristics. However if a nurse does not have these characteristics or value patients as unique individuals, then it is likely that their attitude or approach to patient care is task-centred.

Another important omission from Henderson's (1966) definition is that the unique role of the nurse can only be achieved through nurses working collaboratively with other health care disciplines. Collaboration is not a communication behaviour that nurses (or other health care professionals) are renowned for but it is a communication skill that is essential if nurses are to care for patients in a therapeutic and patient-centred way.

Rutty (1998, p. 249) put forward another view that 'nurses are managers of health who co-ordinate and care for patients'/clients' health throughout their life continuum, both within the acute sector and the community . . . it is the nurse who "knows" the patient and utilizes all the other health care professionals and disciplines in organizing that care.' This is an interesting definition of the role of the nurse because is more specific than Henderson's (1966) and acknowledges that caring for patients is an interdisciplinary process. In using the term 'utilizes' to describe the working relationship between nurses and other health care professionals Rutty (1998) also implied that nurses were superior to all other health professionals and have other disciplines' knowledge and skills at their disposal. By substituting the term 'utilizes' with 'works collaboratively with' Rutty's (1998) definition goes a long way towards defining nursing in a modern context, while at the same time revealing the uniqueness of the nursing role in caring for patients within the health care system. Nurses 'know' the patient better than any other health care worker because they spend time with them and they see the physiotherapists, doctors and occupational therapists come and go. The nurse co-ordinates the contribution of other health care professions to patient care in a way that is therapeutic and patient-centred.

Nurses co-ordinate and provide patient/client care in many different contexts including acute/chronic and community settings. The nurse interprets and translates information for the patient and helps the patient and family derive meaning from the information they receive from other health care disciplines. The nurse communicates between disciplines and across disciplines about patient care and specific patient needs. The nurse does this effectively and successfully because she 'knows' the patient as a person as well as a patient. Figure 8.1 represents a model of nursing within the context of collaborative and patient-centred care.

This model illustrates the context of the nurse–patient relationship in relation to all the other health care disciplines and services. The double arrow indicates that communication between the nurse and patient is two way and collaborative.

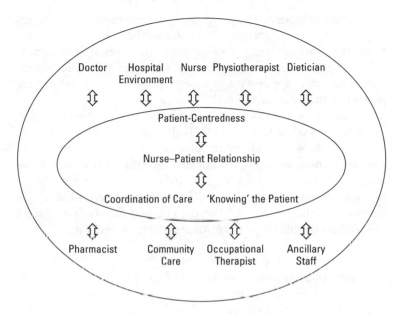

Figure 8.1   A model of nursing within the context of collaborative and patient-centred care

Advocacy

Advocacy is a concept often referred to as an integral aspect of nursing although it could be argued that it is not exclusive to nurses. Advocacy promotes and defends the individualism of patients and is based on an ethical construct. It is essential for all health care professionals (Gadow, 1989; Hewitt, 2002; Llewellyn, 2004). Mallik and McHale (1995) point out that the concept of nurse advocacy is not recognized by law. Advocacy exists in many forms including legal advocacy, self-advocacy, collective advocacy and citizen advocacy (Gates, 1994). A legal advocate is a person who is legally trained and works within legislative frameworks to represent the rights and interests of others. A self-advocate is a person who encourages and helps others to develop confidence and self-esteem. Collective advocacy is when an organization supports a specific group of people. For example, Amnesty International exclusively supports those whose human rights have been violated. Citizen advocacy is probably best known for the support of those with physical and intellectual disabilities. When the parents or guardian of a person with disabilities dies, the state appoints a person who can work with that person in meeting their needs.

An advocate is 'a person who pleads for a cause' (*English Dictionary for Students*, 1999). Blackwell's *Dictionary of Nursing* (1994) described an advocate as 'a person who acts for or defends the rights of another person who is unable or unwilling to act for himself'. A nurse becomes an advocate by being responsible for meeting the patient's needs and through nursing activities done for the patient and family. The rights referred to in this description of an advocate include:

- a right to health care;
- a right to a reasonable standard of care;
- a right to give consent;
- a right of access to health records;
- a right to confidentiality; and
- a right to complain.

(*Source*: Dimond, 1999)

Increasing awareness of their rights means that patients now exercise their rights in questioning doctors and nurses about their treatment and care, making choices about where they get treatment and who gives it and having access to all information relating to their care. Nurses advocate for patients in many ways but perhaps primarily in everyday activities by helping patients make choices that meet their needs; for example how to get out of bed safely, what is the most appropriate food (Llewellyn, 2004). However there are issues for nurses in limiting their ability to carry out the advocacy role. These include the lack of power that nurses have in the context of health care provision. This means that rather than advocating for patients as a group at local or national level, for example in implementing health promotion strategies, nurses are limited to advocating for patients on an individual basis. This too is limited because advocating for a patient can have a negative impact on the nurse. Doctors and other health care disciplines may not like nurses 'interfering' in decisions about patient care. The result is that nurses are often very covert in advocating for patients, particularly in situations where the various health care disciplines do not work collaboratively.

> A nurse accompanies a doctor who tells an elderly patient that he has cancer of the stomach but that the doctors will remove it in an operation. The doctor says that she will return later with the consent form for the patient to sign. The nurse was concerned that the patient had not received enough detail about the surgery or how it would affect the patient's quality of life afterwards so when the doctor had gone, the nurse asked the patient if they understood everything the doctor said. The patient said no and wondered how he would feel after the surgery. The nurse told him that he would have most of his stomach removed in a surgical procedure that would require the patient to spend time in intensive care and he would only be able to eat small amounts of liquidized food in future. Immediately the patient said to the nurse 'I don't want that, I am 78 years old and I like my food. I'd rather continue on the way I am for as long as I can.' The nurse reassured the patient that if that were his decision then he would not have to have surgery. The doctor was very irate when the patient told her he would not give consent for surgery and confronted the nurse who explained that when given the facts, it was the patient's right to decide how he wanted to spend the rest of his life.

This example gives an indication of how the boundaries between advocacy and ethical issues can be blurred and also indicates why the development and use of assertiveness skills is so important in nursing. It would be very difficult and very frustrating for a nurse to advocate for a patient if they could not use assertive skills.

Ethics in nursing

The word 'ethics' is a Greek word that means character and is concerned with systems and behaviour that guide right and wrong. Systems that are ethical are accountable and transparent but yet do not dictate individual human behaviour. Ethics does not provide definitive guidelines for behaviour. Ethical principles related to truth, goodness, justice and freedom form a framework within which ethical issues can be considered. It is the values we hold as human beings that influence the way we live and conduct our lives morally and ethically. This is true also of our role as nurses. Values we hold as nurses and about nursing influence the way we communicate with people and make moral and ethical decisions about their care. Listening, a core communication that was discussed in Chapter 4 lies at the heart of ethics and being ethical and requires commitment, responsibility, attention, reasoning and intelligence on the part of the nurse (Tschudin, 2003). These characteristics and skills are necessary for one to be ethical but also for one to be a nurse that is patient-centred and therapeutic. This takes place within the context of 'knowing the patient' and the uniqueness of nursing within health care practices. This may also be the reason why nurses and doctors can sometimes disagree about patient care. Nursing ethics sometimes conflict with that of other professions because the importance of developing and sustaining the nurse–patient relationship is a fundamental nursing value. Other professions may not understand this because communication between physiotherapists and patients for example is focused on mobility or breathing exercises and is usually transient.

> An 82 year old lady named Elizabeth had an extensive cerebro vascular accident four days ago and is unresponsive. The doctor has said that she should have a PEG tube inserted. The nurse who has been caring for this patient and her family is concerned that this course of treatment is not what the patient or her family would want. Over the previous four days the family had talked about the patient with the nurse. They told her what the lady used to look like, how she liked to dress up and wear her pearls every day and play cards with her friends every Saturday night. She was a great golfer and kept a perfect garden. They expressed enormous sorrow that she would not be able to do these things again and felt that she would not like to live without her independence and quality of life. When the nurse expressed her view that a PEG tube may not be the most appropriate course of treatment for this patient, the doctor was dismissive and said there was no other option. The nurse persisted and suggested that the doctor discuss the issue with the family. The doctor said it had already been discussed with the family who had given their consent. The nurse felt that the family did not fully understand the implications of this course of treatment and talked to the nurse manager. The nurse manager did not agree with the nurse and indicated that she did not wish to continue discussing the matter. The nurse was upset by this and felt that she could not influence the situation.

This is an example of what can happen in reality when nurses regard a particular course of treatment as ethically wrong. The nurse felt that the treatment was futile and served only to prolong the patient's suffering and that as a result of coming to 'know her patient' through the family, this is not what the patient would have wanted. The difference in viewpoint comes from the different values they hold as doctor and nurse and the way in which both professions interpret the ethical aspects of patient care. The outcome of the above interaction is not a positive one and the nurse is left feeling 'let down' by her manager. But this is an example of where there are no right or wrong answers. The doctor, nurse and nurse manager could all justify their views and actions morally and ethically. Junior nurses can find a situation like this particularly difficult and often when faced with the opinions of senior nurses that are based on a different set of personal and professional values, they tend to avoid the situation or remain passive (Kelly, 1998). However this can also occur in nurses who are qualified a number of years, especially if they perceive that they are unsupported by their manager. The outcome of this avoidance and passive behaviour is a feeling of powerlessness and inferiority (Peter *et al.*, 2004).

Exercise

How could the nurse have dealt differently with the situation?

When confronted with opposing views it is important to use assertive behaviour that is confrontational. This is an essential communication skill for the professional development of nurses and Chapter 7 outlines how to be assertive. Remember, being ethical also requires commitment, reasoning and intelligence and this in conjunction with assertive skills means that you do not feel powerless or inferior. Instead you feel that as a nurse, and because you 'know the patient', you are ethically bound to verbalize your concerns regarding their treatment. This type of communication is integral to the development of interdisciplinary collaborative relationships in caring for patients. Working collaboratively does not mean that each discipline (for example, nurses, doctors, physiotherapists) do not have their own agendas. They do, but the patient is at the core of their actions and it is the way in which each member of the health care team communicates and does their work that indicates whether it is ethical and moral or not (Liaschenko and Peter, 2004). The nurse in the scenario above could have persisted even though it would have been difficult for her given the view of her manager and the doctors. By discussing the situation further with the family and establishing whether or not they understood the implications for the patient of inserting a PEG tube, the nurse may have been able to identify issues that needed further discussion. On this basis, dialogue between the doctor and family would need to continue before the tube was inserted with the nurse being more vocal about what was best for the patient as an unique individual.

Professionalism

Nursing has worked hard over the past century to become recognized as a profession. This encompasses characteristics such as an unique body of knowledge, code of ethics, control over work and autonomy in practice to name a few. However not all agree that nursing can or should be a profession because nursing is rooted in practice and by pursuing academic qualifications, nurses would not be as caring towards their patients. Nurses appear to disagree with this view and perceive themselves as intelligent, self-governing and professional especially since the development of specialist and advanced nursing roles (Krebs *et al.*, 1996; Takase *et al.*, 2001).

Traditionally, professions claim to hold ethical values that are demonstrated in codes of professional conduct and have given professions the power to act without reference to external agencies (Colyer, 2004). This level of autonomy was previously the exclusive right of groups such as doctors and lawyers however; with the development of patients' charters and legislation such as the Freedom of Information Act even these groups are required to be more transparent in their accountability. Furthermore, given the consistently fluctuating demands on health care services and the external forces that influence the structure and organization of health care it is difficult for all health care professions to control their work and environment. This means that perhaps autonomy at such a level is no longer realistic, especially within the healthcare context. With the development of numerous professional bodies within health care such as physiotherapy, therapeutic radiography and occupational therapy, medicine is no longer the dominant profession. The question is perhaps not related to whether nursing is a profession or not but rather whether it is equal to others in a health care context. Colyer (2004) suggests that nursing is not equal to other professions, not because nurses do not believe nursing to be equal (and that is an important attribute for any profession) but because of the distorted and stereotypical image of nurses and nursing that is held by the public as a result of media influences. Hart (2004) suggests that image is not that important and the experience of people as patients or consumers is more influential in how nurses are perceived.

The strength of nursing as a profession lies in its ethical basis that values the uniqueness of individuals and patient autonomy above other health care professionals (Redman and Fry, 2000). But for nurses to be recognized as equal by the public within the interdisciplinary delivery of health care they need to communicate as equals. This means communicating assertively, developing negotiating skills and communicating collectively by supporting, respecting and encouraging each other. Working collaboratively with other disciplines also requires these skills. Becoming equal members of the interdisciplinary health care team not just in the delivery of health care at the bedside but also at local and national level in the development and implementation of health care policy and resource allocation requires political behaviour and motivation. As any successful politician knows, effective and positive interpersonal communication is essential in gaining the respect of others. Nurses need to be political and recognize the fundamental importance of positive and effective communication so that they will be instigators of health care reform and successful change agents rather than having change done to them. It is important to remember this will occur within an interdisciplinary context and nurses should be mindful and respectful of other disciplines. For change initiatives and health care services to be patient-focused this process must be collaborative and even though disciplines will still have their own agenda and compete for resources, the focus of all negotiation and communication should be a patient-centred, and high quality interdisciplinary care service. Nurses and nursing are best placed to maintain a patient-centred focus.

Nursing has been described as an art and a science with art representing the unique skilful practice of nursing and science representing knowledge and the provision of evidence to support practice. Nurse theorists and educators have discussed and debated this issue for many years as a means of identifying key elements of nursing that are unique to nursing. Like all health care professions nurses are trying to distinguish themselves from other disciplines, especially medicine, and in doing so attain status and power. Perhaps nursing needs to consider whether this is necessary or appropriate in becoming a profession and recognize that nursing and medicine are interdependent, as are all other health care disciplines when providing care for patients. Conflict is probably inevitable, but as you will have read in Chapter 7, conflict is not the problem; the problem is how to respond to it or manage it successfully. Collaborative communication is the key to managing conflict successfully and is also the key to placing nursing within the interdisciplinary health care team on an equal but distinct footing with other disciplines. Leaders from nursing and medicine should pave the way in developing collaborative working environments, however there is an individual responsibility to communicate collaboratively. This is not just from a nursing perspective, as all health care disciplines need to communicate collaboratively, but for nursing collaborative communication will have a positive impact on the way nursing is viewed by other health care disciplines. As nurses become more political and regarded as equal to other health care professions the public may also change their stereotypical view of nursing.

Accountability

The term accountability has been used in nursing as a means of strengthening its status as a profession and is generally regarded as a key component of professionalism. Walsh (2000, p. 89) describes accountability in nursing as nurses being:

- responsible for their actions at all times;
- able to justify and explain their actions; and
- having the authority to act in the way that they think is best for the patient

Hancock's (1997) argument that nurses do not have the authority to act in a way that they think is best for the patient, and, therefore, cannot be truly accountable is a credible one. According to Hancock (1997) this will not change while current power structures exist within nursing and between nursing and other health care professions. This is an important point not just in relation to accountability but also professionalism, advocacy and autonomy in nursing. Clinical governance provides a framework that could be very useful in bringing about the changes needed to develop a high quality and patient-centred health care service (Walsh, 2000). This is a framework where health care staff are collectively accountable for the quality of patient care. Health care managers and the numerous health care professions work together on the understanding of mutual trust and respect of all involved. This framework embraces and encourages experiential and collaborative learning and development within and between health care professions. The implications of the clinical governance framework for nursing are twofold. The first benefit to nursing is that authority and equality will exist within the context of providing high quality, patient-centred care. The second benefit for nursing and other health care professions is that the power associated with and claimed by medicine will be diluted. Clearly, therefore, the introduction of clinical governance will not be easy and while on paper it seems idealistic to think such a framework can bring about such a radical cultural and organizational change in attitude, the fact that it exists and is proposed at governmental level is most significant.

However, the underlying emphasis on individual responsibility and accountability in the delivery of high quality care and self/professional regulation is perhaps the most significant part of this framework (Wilson, 1998). This recognizes how our personal and professional values regarding the role of the nurse, nursing as a profession and the patient, influence our practice and that without this individual commitment to open, collaborative communication that has the patient's needs at its core, very little will change!

Key points

▶ The values, beliefs and attitudes that a nurse holds about nursing, patients and people generally is reflected in the way they communicate and care for patients.

▶ A nurse's awareness of his/her values helps them identify if the way they communicate is patient-centred or task-centred.

▶ The 'uniqueness' of nursing within healthcare provision lies in 'knowing the patient' and co-ordinating interdisciplinary care. This role needs to be valued and protected by nurses with the context of healthcare development and planning at national and local level.

▶ Collaborative care is essential in providing care that is holistic and patient-centred. Nurses need to embrace this and actively pursue it using political nursing leadership.

▶ In order to be professional, nurses need to be ethical, patient advocates, accountable and autonomous. To do this nurses need to value the work they do as equal members of a collaborative interdisciplinary healthcare team. An essential communication skill in achieving this is assertive behaviour.

9 The role of personal self-awareness in developing therapeutic communication skills

Introduction

While there is a large bulk of literature concerning the whole area of communication, specific research into the role of self-awareness in developing therapeutic communication skills is underdeveloped. Jonathon Rowe in his 1999 paper noted this lack of research in the area. However, he went on to suggest: 'self-awareness can be a significant tool to improve nurse–client interaction and should be an integral part of nurse education'. Based upon the belief in the inherent benefits of being self-aware, Rowe (1999) and others (Betts, 2003; Burnard, 1997) suggested its use in the personal and professional development of nurses. According to Mabe Newman (2003), self-awareness is essential for successful implementation of the therapeutic relationship. Indeed, Betts (2003) considered that a lack of self-awareness contributed to 'communication problems' in nursing. One consideration when exploring the term self-awareness is consideration of its meaning. Kantcheva and Eckroth-Bucher (2002) supported the notion that self-awareness is crucial to the therapeutic nurse–patient relationship. They suggested that to understand another, one must begin with understanding oneself. They also suggested that a lack of self-awareness, or self-understanding, could interfere with the nurse–patient relationship. For example past experiences, attitudes and responses to specific patient populations or circumstances can affect the behaviour of the nurse. Therefore, negative reactions, biases, prejudices and stereotyping must be recognized and explored through self-awareness. Suggested reasons for the development of self-awareness in nurses are outlined in Figure 9.1.

Reasons to develop self-awareness:

- To enhance self-understanding
- To allow acceptance of others
- To become equipped to deal with difficult situations
- To enable self-monitoring
- To enhance personal autonomy

Source: adapted from Burnard, P. (1997) *Know Yourself! Self-Awareness Activities for Nurses and Other Health Professionals*, London: Whurr Publishers Limited.

Figure 9.1   Reasons to develop self-awareness

What is self-awareness?

The *Oxford English Reference Dictionary* (Pearsall and Trumble, 1996) defines self-awareness as 'conscious of one's character, feelings, (and) motives' Burnard (1985, p. 15) described self-awareness as a 'gradual and continuous process of noticing and exploring aspects of self, whether behavioral, psychological or physical with the intention of developing personal and interpersonal understanding'. While consensus regarding definition is not evident, self-awareness as an espoused virtue in nursing refers to the nurse being aware of their verbal and non-verbal behaviours and intentions and how this can impact upon the therapeutic relationship.

 Exercise

Karen, a staff nurse that you are working with, has a tendency to interrupt when people are speaking to her.
   Can you think what message this may send to patients unintentionally?
   Can you identify ways that Karen could become aware of this habit?

You may have suggested that the patient may interpret this interrupting in a negative way, perhaps sensing anger or frustration from the nurse. You may have suggested that a peer review of Karen's role may reveal this tendency to interrupt or you may have suggested reflection. Reflection is gaining increasing popularity within the nursing profession. Indeed, it is espoused that nurses become reflective practitioners. Methods such as this for increasing self-awareness will be considered later in the chapter. However, the meaning of 'self' and 'self-awareness' require some discussion in the interim.

Awareness

Awareness is often described as a human feature. Unlike animals, humans, through consciousness, are aware of themselves, their thoughts, feelings, behaviour and physical and emotional self. Self-awareness is the ability to perceive one's own existence, including feelings and behaviours; it is a personal understanding of one's identity. At a basic level, each human has an awareness of self. There is a consciousness and awareness of those aspects of self as described in Figure 9.2. However, within nursing self awareness has become associated with a developmental process of getting to know the self more. A key author in this area, Burnard (1992, 1997) highlighted the increased development of self-awareness as a positive element in nurses and a requirement of professional

---

Burnard's (1997) Model of Self

- The physical aspect of self
- The real self
- The ideal self
- The self-for-others
- The social self
- The spiritual self
- The darker aspect of self
- The sexual self

Source: adapted from Burnard, P. (1997) *Know Yourself! Self-Awareness Activities for Nurses and Other Health Professionals*, London: Whurr Publishers Limited.

Figure 9.2   Burnard's (1997) Model of Self

nursing practice. Burnard (1997, p. 25) described self-awareness as 'a continous and evolving process of getting to know who you are'. While humans by their very nature possess an awareness of self, it is held that the elements of self can be explored and developed in order to improve communication skills (Burnard, 1997).

Self

There is a significant body of psychological literature that examines the concept of self. Ellis and Gates (2003) highlighted that theorists are often divided on their interpretations and understandings of self, awareness and consciousness. Psychological theorists who explore the nature of self and are commonly associated with communication in nursing include Sigmund Freud and Carl Rogers (1961) (see Chapter 3). Freud proposed the notion of the unconscious self, whereby individual's reactions to situations may be unconscious and linked to past experience such as childhood. A number of unconscious defence mechanisms are also outlined, such as denial, repression, displacement and reaction formation. Self-awareness is not referred to explicitly within this theory. As self-awareness requires self-consciousness, the unconscious nature of individuals as proposed by Freud, with complex ego defence mechanisms, warrant self-exploration – a difficult and highly specialized task, possibly requiring professional assistance.

Behaviourism on the other hand oversimplifies the human condition, reducing it to one of response to stimulus from the external environment. Human self-awareness and self-consciousness are restricted as we are reactors rather than being in control of our own behaviours (Ellis and Gates, 2003).

The humanistic model pays greater attention to self-awareness. Rogers (1961) asserted that humans are dynamic reactive individuals who seek to achieve their full potential. Humans are motivated towards continual self-improvement.

Peplau (1991) described how the self develops from appraisals made by self and significant others about self, as an infant and child. Continued repeating of these appraisals become a pattern that is incorporated into self. With each new era of development, the self may be reappraised. Thus Peplau (1991) asserts that the development of self is an ongoing process that continues throughout life.

Burnard (1997) provided a simple model of self. Using this model the self may be conceptualized as containing multiple and interrelated aspects of self that come together to form a whole (Figure 9.2).

Burnard (1997, p. 7) describes the physical self as the '*bodily* sense of self' (emphasis author's own). He suggested that communication occurs 'through our physical sense of self', that is through non-verbal communication which he described as 'body language' (Burnard, 1997, p. 7). These means include eye contact, touch, gesture, proximity to others, and non-verbal aspects of speech and facial expression.

Burnard (1997, p. 9) described the real self as one that is personal and not usually known by a wide circle of acquaintances. It is essentially private and described as 'internal'. Burnard (1997) suggested that aspects of this often hidden dimension of people contains common items; that people share hidden aspects of self that often are common to many people, but not necessarily disclosed. Burnard (1997) also argued that perhaps there is no real self, but that we play out a series of roles in our lives. Our real self is little more than a 'collection of scripts and roles that we acquire over the years of our life' (Burnard, 1997, p. 10).

The ideal self, he suggested is the 'day dream about how we would like to be' (Burnard, 1997, p. 11). This may originate from ideas that we have about how others live their lives. The ideal self is therefore a 'picture in our heads' (Burnard, 1997). The self for others is those aspects of self that we present to others and is dependent upon our relationship with them. The social self relates to how we present ourselves in groups. The spiritual self is described as 'often associated with religion, (but) it need not necessarily be so' (Burnard, 1997, p. 15). Burnard equated it with individuals seeking meaning and purpose in their lives. Burnard contended that this is another very personal aspect of the self that sometimes people do not wish to discuss. The darker self, Burnard suggests relates to the 'skeletons in the cupboard' (1997, p. 19). These may be aspects of the self that 'we do not particularly like' (1997,

p. 19). These include: aggressive feelings towards others, sexual thoughts and thoughts and feelings that we perceive to be unusual to ourselves and not necessarily shared by others.

With regard to the sexual self, Burnard described two distinct aspects: the sexual orientation and the sexual identity. The latter refers to whether an individual is male or female and the former refers to the sexual orientation. Expression of sexuality within sexual orientation, Burnard (1997) suggested, could occur in many ways including: heterosexual orientation (expression of sexual attraction to persons of the opposite sex), homosexual (expression of sexual attraction to persons of the same sex), and bisexual (expression of sexual attraction to persons of both the same and opposite sex).

Communication models for increasing self-awareness

A move away from ritualistic and task-based nursing is required to encourage nurses away from the use of linear models of communication. These latter models focus on the basic principles of communication (message–sender–receiver) and although the message may be communicated, there is little consideration of the relationship. Chapter 3 also identified partnership as an important theme in the contemporary use of conceptual models of nursing (Pearson *et al.*, 2000). The development of the nurse–patient relationship was identified as crucial to this process (Orem, 2001). When non-linear models of communication are used, such as the Comforting Interaction-Relationship Model (Morse *et al.*, 1997) the therapeutic relationship becomes increasingly important. There is an unconscious nature to this interaction, as referred to in Chapter 3 and this suggests an unawareness of our personal contribution to the interaction.

Relatives in O'Shea's (2004) study found that recognition and a wave by nurses that had previously nursed their infant held significant value for them in the hospital environment. Simiarly, Astedt-Kurki and Haggman-Laitila (1992) and Williams (1998) found that the words and body language that nurses chose to use when approaching patients affected the extent to which communication was patient-centred. Timmins *et al.* (2005) highlighted that small behaviours have potentially great impact across a variety of nursing situations, and suggested that small gestures can make a difference. Griffiths (Timmins *et al.*, 2005) termed these 'microbehaviors', which have increased significance in situations where individuals have cognitive dysfunction.

However, the challenge remains for nurses to examine these microbehaviours to ascertain their impact on the development of the therapeutic relationship with patients. While nurse communication texts have typically drawn upon psychological theories that explain and predict behaviour, preferred models for the development of self-awareness have traditionally been a rather simplified version of these. Burnard (1997) for example suggested the use of the Johari Window, originally developed by Luft (1969) (Figure 9.3).

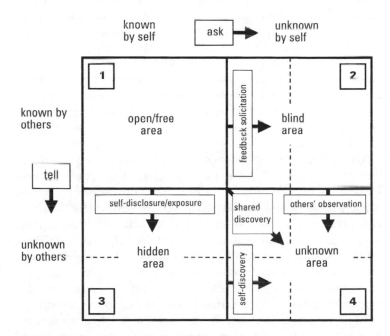

Figure 9.3 Johari Window Model

In this model a window represents a person. The 'open' quadrant represents things that one knows about oneself, and others also know. This is also known as the free area (Chapman, 2005). The 'blind' quadrant represents things that others may know about a person, but that person is unaware of. The 'hidden' quadrant represents things one know about oneself, that others do not know. The 'unknown' quadrant represents things that neither the person nor others knows about that person. This model allows for use of psychological theories as mentioned earlier. The unknown quadrant could refer to Freud's unconscious reactions or defence mechanisms, or to behaviourist responses to the environment. Rogers (1961) suggested that some degree of self-disclosure benefits relationships and increases self-esteem. However, psychology is a highly specialized field and an analysis of self may require professional assistance. Indeed, Rowe (1999) suggested that Johari Window use requires a 'trained, experienced facilitator' although professional assistance wasn't espoused by other writers that referred to this model (Burnard, 1997).

The basic concept of the Johari Window is to examine hidden selves through disclosure and feedback from others about our blind area. These processes of disclosure and feedback can enhance the sense of self, and promote self-awareness. This is rather like the process described by Burnard (1997).

Other methods to promote self-awareness have been put forward by ASTD (American Society for Training and Development). Founded in 1944, ASTD professes to be the world's largest association dedicated to workplace learning and performance professionals. Elaine Siciliano wrote on the subject of self-awareness for their Dallas chapter (Siciliano, 2005). She suggested that self-awareness is 'reading one's own emotions and recognizing their impact'. She suggests that through self-awareness and recognition of emotions valuable information can be learned. She also supports the notion of building personal strength from acknowledging 'weakness'. Methods of developing self-awareness that she suggested were asking others for feedback, engaging a coach to review your strengths and weaknesses, taking personality tests (such as those found on Queendom.com, 2005). Another suggestion is to develop a list of situations at work that sparked emotional reactions or were difficult to resolve. Write a few sentences for each situation describing what happened, how you felt, what you said, what the other person said, how it turned out. Through this writing, themes and possible triggers can be identified to help modify reactions in similar situations in the future. Other suggestions included setting aside a half hour daily for prayer and/or keeping a journal to record insights, feelings, and daily situations.

Benefits of self-awareness

In the UK, the NHS Modernization Agency Leadership Centre (2005) provided guidance on leadership development. This organization stated that self-awareness is a core component of the development of good leadership skills. They suggested that self-awareness could be a very useful skill for leaders of health care to develop. Leadership is a valuable skill for nurses at all levels, and is an essential skill of practicing nurses. They suggested that developing knowledge of personal strengths and limitations through increased self-awareness could assist with understanding one's own emotions and the impact of one's behaviour on others. They identified a measurement scale for assessing personal levels of self-awareness as component of the leadership qualities frame-work (Figure 9.4).

The NHS Modernization Agency Leadership Centre (2005) also suggested that a high level of self-awareness, as identified from Figure 9.4, helps sustain the leaders' energy and resilience, enabling them to deal with difficult situations. Another benefit of self-awareness development is the ability to learn from mistakes or misjudgements and this is a prevalent theme in the self-awareness literature. They also suggested that by recognizing their own strengths and limitations managers are more likely to empower others. 'Successful collaborative working requires leaders who are well aware of, and sensitive to, the impact they have on others in a range of work situations' (The NHS Modernization Agency Leadership Centre, 2005).

---

0 **Fails to consider own emotions**

- Does not stop to understand own emotions.
- May be surprised by own reactions to certain situations; and does not set time aside for personal reflection.
- Does not recognize or acknowledge the impact of own behaviour on others.

1 **Registers own emotions**

- Is aware of their own feelings.
- Notices when their emotions are aroused.

2 **Understands own emotions**

- Understands the nature and causes of their emotional reactions to particular situations.
- Recognizes how challenges to their personal values are likely to trigger certain responses in them.

3 **Understands own strengths and limitations**

- Understands the likely implications and impact of their emotions, both on self and others in a range of situations.
- Knows their own strengths, and limitations, in providing leadership that makes a difference to patients and users.

Source: NHS Modernization Agency Leadership Centre Leadership Qualities Framework (LQFR); online at: www.executive.modern.nhs.uk/framework/personalqualities/selfawareness.aspex Crown Copyright with permission.

Figure 9.4 Levels of self-awareness

Burnard (1997) also suggested ways in which self-awareness may be important in nursing (Figure 9.5). It must be noted however that these benefits are merely proposed and little empirical research has been carried out in this area. What is of interest to note from Figure 9.5 is that while self-awareness is a personal journey, the professed benefits are primarily the assistance of others. There are issues with this trajectory. First, there is little evidence confirming that the development of self-awareness can improve performance as little or no experimental work has been carried out on the topic. Second, with an emphasis on highlighting both strengths and weak-

Proposed benefits from self-awareness

- Ensuring that people feel cared for
- Understanding other people's needs and wants
- Helping people express their feelings
- Coping with other people's pain
- Helping with people who are dying
- Helping the bereaved
- Working with children
- Learning nursing
- Doing research
- Understanding your colleagues
- Learning to relax
- Getting on better with your friends and family
- Planning your work
- Identifying your strengths and deficits
- Planning your future
- Identifying your learning needs
- Organizing the work of others

Source: adapted from Burnard, P. (1997) *Know Yourself! Self-Awareness Activities for Nurses and Other Health Professionals*, London: Whurr Publishers Limited.

Figure 9.5   Proposed benefits from self-awareness

nesses, there may be a tendency for some to focus upon weaknesses rather than strengths. One example is when nursing students are writing journals, diaries or reflective pieces of writing there is a tendency to reflect upon negative experiences, as these tend to stand out more, and perhaps the benefit of reflecting upon good experiences is not clear. Developing self-awareness has become synonymous with reflection, which has gained increasing popularity in nursing over the past 20 years.

Reflection

Reflection is a recurring theme in nursing literature (Hannigan, 2001). Based upon the work of Dewey (1933), Schön (1983) and others, reflection has become an espoused activity in nursing and nurse education in both the UK and Europe (Burns and Bulman, 2000). The recent UK *Fitness for*

Practice report on the initial education of nurses reaffirmed support for the idea of the reflective practitioner, declaring that students should be able to 'demonstrate critical awareness and reflective practice' (United Kingdom Central Council for Nursing Midwifery and Health Visiting (UKCC), 1999, p. 38). A similar belief in the intrinsic value of reflection exists in other countries such as the Republic of Ireland where all nursing graduates are expected to be reflective practitioners (Government of Ireland, 2000). Thus learning outcomes related to reflection have become a component part of many undergraduate nurse education programmes and reflection forms the basis for many formative assessments (Hannigan, 2001). Carroll *et al.* (2002) were critical of both the teaching and assessment of reflection and reflective practice in nursing, suggesting that 'the literature on reflection and reflective practice is sparse in terms of research evidence. Large amounts of descriptive anecdotal literature exist, but conclusive answers to the question of what is reflection and how it is to be taught/learned are not apparent.' One concern expressed by these authors was the lack of empirical evidence with regard to improvement in patient outcome with the use of reflection. This argument was supported in a commentary on the paper written by Newell (2002), a seminal author on the topic. Newell supported the argument that reflection may be a topic that is nebulous and not fully articulated or examined, with little purported benefits to patients ultimately emerging. These criticisms need to be borne in mind when considering reflection in the context of practice and the development of reflective practice, which is another concept entirely, again not fully elucidated. That said however, there is potential for self-development from using the processes of reflection to think back over one's actions and to commit those memories to paper, rendering them easier to analyse and thus learn from. Hannigan (2001) did caution however against a mechanistic view of reflection, which is a comment often received from nursing students. The process should be dynamic and cyclical. Johns (1999) suggested that guided reflection can be emancipatory and a powerful tool within nursing. Johns (1999) also raised the question as to whether reflection should be a solitary operation or used with guidance. Traditionally within nursing this has been an individual occupation. However, this may be dependent upon purpose. For the purpose of self-development, using the Johari Window framework, the use of another person is helpful to provide feedback that is crucial in developing awareness. Indeed the notion of reflection has been criticized for being too introspective, and failing to take into account the wider health care perspective (Brechin *et al.*, 2000). By focusing solely on what the individual thinks and feels in a given situation there is a tendency towards personal bias and missing out on vital information.

There are several models of reflection on action cited in the literature, such as Johns (1999) and Gibbs (1988). These models stimulate reflection after an event has taken place. The focus is upon analysing the situation, exploring feelings, behaviours and reactions, and learning from that experience. Strategies used to promote reflection among nursing students include analysis of critical incidents, diaries and journals (Hannigan, 2001). Jensen and Joy (2005) in their analysis of junior baccalaureate nursing students' journals found very little evidence of reflection taking place. However, of all journal entries, 18 per cent were at higher levels, and 82 per cent were at lower levels. There are several issues and omissions to be considered with the use of reflection. First, the overall benefits to nursing care from the use of reflection are debatable (Newell, 2002).

While there are professed benefits to using models of reflection, there is little empirical evidence that indicates personal or professional benefits (Carroll *et al.*, 2002). Reflection may be overly introspective (Brechin, 2000) and not contain the essential element of feedback from others that is required to develop self awareness. While personal reflection remains internalized there is always the risk of defence mechanisms coming into play and as Burnard (1997) describes these can be used to 'fool' ourselves.

For example a nursing student may realize through reflection that more communication and explanation could have been afforded to the client during a procedure (for example while providing an intramuscular injection). Although the student admits this, through the course of reflection, the student may use rationalization and intellectualization to provide excuses for the behaviour and thus justify it. The student may decide that little change in the said behaviour is required. As long as reflection remains personal this risk will be there. Alternative solutions are guided reflection, as suggested by Johns (1999), or expanding reflection techniques to encompass critical practice.

Barnett (1997) suggested that inherent domains of critical practice are critical analysis, critical action and critical reflexivity. It is argued that health professionals require all three skills to meet the challenges of a practice that is filled with uncertainty (Brechin, 2000). *Critical analysis* requires on-going enquiry and analysis. Rather than simply relying upon prior knowledge and policies, the practitioner *evaluates* their relevance. As opposed to an individualistic perspective, critical analysis recognizes multiple perspectives. *Critical action* requires a sound knowledge base, but seeks to address power differences, and *critical reflexivity* requires a practitioner who is self-aware in his/her practice. Critical practice is viewed as a process. Further exploration of these domains serves to illuminate the potential contribution of these concepts to nursing practice.

Critical analysis

Critical practice is represented by an overlap of critical analysis, critical action and critical reflexivity (Barnett, 1997). The specific components of critical analysis are outlined in Figure 9.6.

Evaluation of knowledge, theories, policy, and practice

Recognition of multiple perspectives

Different levels of analysis

Ongoing enquiry

Source: adapted from Brechin, A. (2000) Introducing critical practice. In A. Brechin, H. Brown and M. Eby (eds), *Critical Practice in Health and Social Care*, London: Sage Publications, 25–47.

Figure 9.6 Key features of critical analysis

Using critical analysis as a reflective framework can encourage you to question your practice. You may begin to examine inherent strengths and weaknesses of your practice. You can evaluate current knowledge and theory and the analysis will be continuous and ongoing and occur at multiple levels. It will also occur at personal level. You can continuously question your own knowledge and theory base to evaluate the extent to which it informs current practice.

Increasingly the nursing profession is also being called upon to recognize different perspectives. Modern health care strategies require a people-centred approach, where the consumer (i.e., the patient) is placed at the centre of health care. Rather than nursing priorities as the centre of care, critical analysis encourages nurses to see the patient perspective.

Critical action

The key features of critical action can be viewed in Figure 9.7. Critical practice also requires a solid skill base. Critical action requires empowering the nursing profession from within. Improving knowledge and skills through continuous education and development is one element. Empowerment of patients also involves tackling some of the oppression that exists within society towards marginalized groups (Pinkery, 2000).

Sound skill base used with awareness of context
Operating to challenge structural disadvantage
Working with difference towards empowerment

Source: adapted from Brechin, A. (2000) Introducing critical practice. In A. Brechin, H. Brown and M. Eby (eds), *Critical Practice in Health and Social Care*, London: Sage Publications, 25–47.

Figure 9.7   Key features of critical action

Engaged self
Negotiated understanding and interventions
Questioning personal values and assumptions

Source: adapted from Brechin, A. (2000) Introducing critical practice. In A. Brechin, H. Brown and M. Eby (eds), *Critical Practice in Health and Social Care*, London: Sage Publications, 25–47.

Figure 9.8 Key features of critical reflexivity

Critical reflexivity

The impetus for and the origin of both critical analysis and critical action are largely outside the individual (Brechin, 2000). The professional role and the organization provide an incentive and a platform for these activities, and indeed a certain responsibility exists therein. However, the third aspect of critical practice, critical reflexivity, is inherently personal. The key features of critical reflexivity can be viewed in Figure 9.8. Reflexivity is a particularly useful skill for developing self-awareness. Critical reflexivity provides direction for you to think about practice. While reflection in isolation has been criticized for being too individualistic within health care delivery, critical reflexivity within the context of critical practice is not. The guiding principles of critical practice are 'respecting others as equals' and 'adopting a not-knowing approach' (Brechin, 2000, pp. 31, 32). Analysing policy, challenging oppression and introspection must be done with respect. The approach should be objective. Adopting a not-knowing approach is the only feasible option open to today's nurses and all practitioners.

Developing professional confidence

The discussion of self-awareness within the nursing context focuses upon the recognition of personal strengths and weakness. To a certain extent the personal weaknesses are the focus of scrutiny as the nurse seeks to improve behaviour that will ultimately help the therapeutic relationship. While the use of critical practice as a model for self-development is less focused on the person and less likely, therefore, to focus upon weaknesses, the impact of disclosure on individuals needs consideration. In the absence of guided reflection described by Johns (1999), the nursing student runs the risk of first applying defence mechanisms during reflection (rationalization, intellectualization, projection, reaction formation, suppression, repression, regression) or conversely actually internalizing negative findings that could possibly reduce confidence. The use of a professional guide, such as a counsellor or facilitator would reduce this risk as the person could be coached away from this line of thinking. However, something that is not often considered when reviewing this topic is improving professional confidence rather than instilling values and beliefs around a mistake culture. Unlike self-awareness and reflection, the concept of confidence is something that has undergone significantly theoretical and empirical development under the guidance of Bandura (1977).

Bandura (1977) introduced the term self-efficacy as the personally held belief in one's own ability to execute a task successfully. Expectations of personal efficacy are based on four major sources of information: past performance accomplishments, past experience, verbal persuasion, and physiological states (Bandura 2000). Confidence or self-efficacy differs from self-esteem, which, according to Grainger (1990), is an intrinsic feeling of self-worth and self-respect. She sites intrinsic factors affecting self-confidence in nursing as the presence of knowledge and ability. Extrinsic factors include the public or nurses' view of nursing and the way the managers, peers, and other professionals react to the nurse. Davidhizar (1993, p. 218) suggests the following definition: 'Self-confidence is the feeling that someone knows how to do something, has the power to make things happen, and knows that one's efforts will be successful; it is the belief that knowledge, skill, experience, and potential will result in success.'

According to Bandura (1997) this self-efficacy makes a difference in how people feel, think and act. For example, a low sense of self-efficacy is associated with depression, anxiety, and helplessness (Scholz *et al.*, 2002). The latter may result in low self-esteem and negative views of one's personal accomplishments and personal development. Conversely, a high self-efficacy improves performance including that of decision-making and academic achievement (Scholz *et al.*, 2002). Therefore, self-efficacy levels can improve or reduce motivation. People with high self-efficacy often choose to perform more challenging tasks (Bandura, 1997). They often set high goals that they are determined to achieve (Schwarzer and Schmitz, 2004). High self-efficacy also allows them to recover quickly from setbacks that occur, therefore maintaining commitment to their original goals (Schwarzer and Schmitz, 2004). Thus self-efficacy allows individuals to explore and respond to challenging environments (Scholz *et al.*, 2002).

Scholz *et al.* (2002) suggested that self-efficacy is 'domain-specific'. This means that firm self-beliefs can be held in particular situations or levels of functioning. For example, a person may have a high self-efficacy in one area such as academic achievement; but it may be low in the area of relationships. However a more global and generalized sense of self-efficacy was also described referring to confidence in one's coping ability across a wide range of demanding or novel situations (Bandura, 2000). General self-efficacy refers to broad personal competence to deal effectively with a variety of situations. According to Bandura's (1986) social cognitive theory, individuals possess a self-system that enables them to exercise a certain degree of control over their thoughts, feelings, motivations and actions (Pajares, 1997).

Bandura (1986) suggested that, through the process of self-reflection, individuals are able to evaluate their experiences and thought processes (Pajares, 1997). As a result personal knowledge, skills and accomplishments don't always necessarily predict future attainments as beliefs about capabilities powerfully influence all future behaviours (Pajares, 1997). Behaviour is influenced not only by previous performances but also by self-efficacy beliefs as a result of reflection (Pajares, 1997). Thus reflection alone is not sufficient to improve performance. It could indeed have a negative effect. For example, a nursing student who reflects upon a skill performed and judges it to be poor, may have a low self-efficacy related to this skill for the future. Thus a supportive environment with the use of a facilitator would be most helpful in the development of student reflections in these areas and future confidence with nursing skills. Bandura (2000) identified observing mastery in others and role modelling as important aspects of developing self-efficacy. This provides a supportive environment wherein a person can develop under supervision. Nursing students should, where possible, aim to develop self-awareness skills under the guidance of a facilitator, preceptor, mentor, teacher or guide as appropriate. Johns (1999) did question the absolute requirement for reflection to be a solitary operation and suggested the possible use of guidance. Furthermore one analysis of nursing students' reflections observed little or no evidence of reflection having taken place (Jensen and Joy, 2005).

Increasingly professional reflection is being suggested to occur in the wider context of the health care environment, rather than on an individual basis (Brechin, 2000). Reflection, which may be utilized to develop both self-awareness and self-efficacy, is a useful tool for nursing students and practicing nurses that could be used with guidance. Moreover, critical practice, which subsumes reflection, is considered an alternative way forward for developing self-awareness and reflexivity.

Key points

▶ Self-awareness is an essential ingredient in the development of effective patient-centred communication. It is also essential for personal and, therefore, professional growth and development.

▶ Self-awareness is about knowing and understanding ourselves and without it we cannot begin to understand others.

▶ Developing self-awareness requires that our feelings, actions, values, attitudes and beliefs are brought into our consciousness and we become aware of how we as individuals and nurses influence our relationships and interactions with others.

▶ Critical analysis, critical action and critical reflexivity are considered essential factors in developing professional self-awareness and are the key components of critical practice.

10 Experiential learning

Introduction

Securing and practicing from a uniform knowledge base is essential to the development of the discipline of nursing. It is widely recognized and accepted that nursing practice must be research-based. Internationally, the use of research in nursing is regarded as a necessary step in an age of continued rapid technological development and quality care. Increasingly, practitioners are called upon to justify their practice, and ensure that it is based on sound evidence. What constitutes evidence attracts debate within the nursing domain; and research is an accepted and legitimate source of evidence that is essential for many aspects of nursing care.

However, the research base for nurse–patient communication and the development of the therapeutic relationship with clients is not well established. While textbooks on communication abound, most of the work is prescriptive and descriptive, thus describing models of communication and outlining how nurses in practice may use these. As outlined in Chapter 1, many of these conceptual models fail to fully account for the complexity of the communication process, and while these models may be useful for developing an understanding of aspects of communication, they provide little by way of direction for nurse–patient communication in the clinical setting. Although they serve to provide some explanation for communication events they are abstract and removed from the dynamic interaction of communication within the therapeutic relationship. Chapter 1 also highlighted how few of these theories are specific to nursing. Morse *et al.* (1992) developed a model of communication that focuses on the emotional engagement of the nurse with the patient (Figure 1.2). The model is based on two key characteristics. The first is whether the nurse is patient-focused or nurse-focused and the second is whether the communication is spontaneous (first-level) or learned (second-level). Fosbinder (1994) revealed that important aspects of communication from patients' perspectives were translating, getting to know you, establishing trust and going the extra mile. Morse *et al.* (1992) also highlighted the importance of the display of sympathy by nurses to patients. McCabe (2004) in her study supported this finding.

Morse *et al.* (1997) developed the Comforting Interaction-Relationship Model and identified three components of communication: nursing actions, patient actions and the evolving relationship. Nursing actions consist of comforting strategies, styles of care and nursing patterns of relating. Patient actions consist of signals of discomfort, indices of distress and patterns of relating to a nurse. The evolving relationship is the third component of this model and it describes nursing and patient actions as the means by which the nurse–patient relationship is negotiated by the nurse and patient and subsequently develops. Nurses respond to patient signals of discomfort and indices of distress using comforting strategies, styles of caring and patterns of relating on an ongoing and changing basis.

Nurses often use a linear model of one-way communication in the practice setting (sender–message–receiver) that limits communication and the development of the nurse–patient relationship (Bradley and Edinberg, 1990; Kruijver *et al.*, 2001). It is suggested that *principles* of good communication, such as those suggested by Morse *et al.* (1997), rather than nurses in the health care setting using static models of communication, results in more effective patient-centred communication.

The use of conceptual models and research evidence as the primary informant of nursing practice has received criticism from scholars who hold postmodern views. Several contemporary authors contend that current theories of nursing and models of nursing are inadequate to inform the complexity of healthcare situations (Marks-Maran, 1999; Spitzer, 1998a, b). Postmodern rejection of theories of nursing, models of nursing and the use of the Nursing Process stem from the postmodern rejection of 'grand theories' to inform practice. 'Postmodernism challenges the modernist idea of a single transcendent meaning of reality and the importance of the search for empirical patterns that correspond to and represent ultimate meaning' (Reed, 1995, p. 3). The concern of those with postmodern views is that the individual meaning and context of each situation has relevance and importance rather than subscribing to the notion that 'one model fits all' (Timmins, 2002).

Under the current, mainly positivistic paradigm, Spitzer (1998b) suggests that, 'nursing has difficulties in highlighting to both patients and the system where nursing can and does make a difference.' The postmodern era is characterized by pluralism, variety and contingency where positivistic beliefs in science, truths, objectivity and certainty are undermined (Mitchell, 1996).

Lay knowledge emerges as an important concept (Mitchell, 1996). From a nursing perspective, this implies that patients need greater involvement in their care, including patient assistance in the use and selection of models of nursing (Graeme, 2000). It could also include eclectic choice of the nursing model (Lister, 1997) or building on established theory using the ideas and views of nurses locally, in order to develop a model for use (Graeme, 2000; Mitchell, 1996).

A further notion is the development and exploration of nursing knowledge using interpretive approaches (Benner, 1984, 1999; Parton, 1994). Rather than using frameworks that involve listing diagnoses and matching interventions, (static models), Benner *et al.*, (1999) suggested that the practice of critical care nursing should expand the boundaries of current theory and models of nursing because of the inherent complexity of the environment. Interventions are instantaneous and highly context-dependent. As an alternative, these authors suggest that critical care nurses should focus on six aspects of clinical judgement and skillful behaviour: (1) reasoning-in-transition; (2) skilled knowledge; (3) response-based practice; (4) agency; (5) perceptual ability and the skill of involvement; and (6) the links between clinical and ethical reasoning. These aspects of practice may serve as a guide for use within each of the domains of practice that they identify, to articulate nursing care for documentation and teaching and improving practice (Benner *et al.*, 1999).

A similar approach could be used with communication. Nursing actions (comforting strategies, styles of care and nursing patterns of relating) described by Morse *et al.* (1992) could be used as a framework within which to develop a repertoire of communication skills. Through ongoing reflection on practice, including feedback from both clients and peers, nursing actions, patient actions and the evolving relationship could be articulated. Rather than expecting a communication model or theory to fully inform practice, the nurse may develop a dynamic theory through critical practice. This complies with Watson's (1999) notion of a science of caring that embraces 'inquiries that are reflective, subjective and interpretative as well as objective-empirical' (Watson, 2005). Watson suggested that this caring science served as an 'intellectual blueprint for nursing's evolving disciplinary/professional matrix, rather than a specific theory per se'. To this end it is useful to incorporate some of her principles here.

Watson (2005) advocated multiple approaches to inquiry and theory building including clinical and empirical approaches, but was also open to moving other areas of inquiry such as the aesthetic, poetic and narratives. Thus in a postmodern era, there is a place for building upon theory using reflection, narratives, personal enquiry and experiential learning.

Methods of experiential learning in communication

Communication with patients and clients takes place in many environments, hospital wards and clinics, nursing homes and clients' own homes. The nursing student, although equipped with the relevant classroom preparation and theory is likely to learn a great deal about communication through a variety of experiences. In order to draw out specific learning from those experiences it may be helpful to begin to write up a daily journal or diary, or simply write about critical incidents or those interactions that may have struck you as important in some way during the day. Diaries are often used in nursing and are mostly for the personal use of the student. Writing is free from restrictions, and is a personal narrative, however to preserve confidentiality of patients and clients, names and other identifiable characteristics should be avoided when making references to practice. Security of the diary/journal is also important, and it should be kept in a safe and private place at all times. This journal or diary would represent a narrative giving a descriptive account of one's experiences of the practice of nursing. It may be useful for articulating and clarifying thoughts and facilitate the development of questions about practice that may be investigated through one's course of study or by subsequently asking questions of a mentor/ preceptor or staff nurse.

> Katie is a first year student nurse working on a cardiac ward. She begins writing her diary on her first day of the placement on the ward and writes it up each evening. She is four weeks on the ward and is getting used to performing in this environment. However, she realized from writing her diary last evening that there are still several items in the morning report/handover that she does not understand. This relates particularly to abbreviations used by staff. She decides to ask a member of staff to talk through the report with her at a quiet period the following day.

This example demonstrates how a simple description of the day's activities revealed an item that Katie needed to address. This type of work is personal and superficial. In order to deepen the level of analysis the use of a model of reflection such as Gibbs *et al.* (1994) may be used.

Using a model of reflection

Using a model of reflection such as Gibbs *et al.* (1994) provides a little more structure than a diary or journal. It provides specific guidelines and direction for the thought processes. This can be used on a specific topic or incident being discussed within a diary or journal, or it can be performed as an isolated reflection exercise. It is useful to use the steps of the cycle of reflection as subheadings to describe and analyse the situation. The subheadings are outlined in Figure 10.1.

Steps in Reflection

- Description: what happened?
- Feelings: what were you thinking/feeling?
- Evaluation: what was good and bad about the experience?
- Conclusion: what else would you have done?
- Analysis: what sense can you make of the situation?
- Action Plan: if it arose again what would you do?

Source: adapted fromn Gibbs, G., Palmer, A., Burns, S. and Bulman, C. (1994) *Reflective Practice in Nursing*, Oxford: Blackwell Scientific Publications.

Figure 10.1   Steps in the reflection process

An example of a reflection is outlined below.

Description: What happened?

On the ward today I was asked whether I would like to give an injection to a patient. I had seen it being given before but hadn't done one yet.

Feelings: what were you thinking/feeling?

I was delighted that I was getting a chance to do it. They don't come up that often in this ward

Evaluation: what was good and bad about the experience?

The staff nurse who supervised me explained everything in advance and that was great. I really felt confident when I began. I gave the injection pretty well I think, the nurse said that I had done well.

Conclusion: what else would you have done?

Although actually giving the injection went well, I don't think that I focused enough on the patient. The nurse did all the talking and explaining as I was so focused on what I was doing. Looking back on it, I could have explained things more to the patient and involved her a little more.

Analysis: what sense can you make of the situation?

I mentioned these thoughts to the nurse afterwards, and she explained that as I was a junior student, and it was my first time, this was not unusual. I agree with this, it was very difficult to come to grips with holding all the equipment, positioning myself and trying to explain things to the patient at the same time. I suppose this will improve with time.

Action Plan: if it arose again what would you do?

Definitely, even as a junior student I would make a bigger effort to provide explanations to the patient.

Using a model such as Gibbs *et al.* (1994) provides structure and guidelines for reflection and can guide the student towards future action in the area. Criticisms of model use include the tendency for students to focus on negative aspects of their practice, or to search for negative aspects. This may be as a result of the subheadings which, while useful, are also leading. The last section for example 'what would you do if it arose again?', and 'what else could you have done?' may lead the student to look for situations where action is needed (as opposed to no action being required). There is also a tendency for this type of reflection to be self-limiting. It is a superficial analysis of subjective feelings on an event and it is unclear whether this is useful or meaningful to students or whether (as described in Chapter 9) it has any overall impact upon nursing practice.

One method of advancing reflection and experiential learning is critical practice (Chapter 9). Rather than providing an introspective analysis, Barnett's (1997) model of critical practice encourages feedback from others and consideration of the context in which the practice of nursing takes place.

Critical analysis requires on going enquiry and analysis. Rather than simply relying upon prior knowledge and policies, the practitioner *evaluates* their relevance. Using the example of the administration of an intramuscular injection above, the student, when engaging in critical analysis, would not only explore personal feelings and behaviours, but move outside of this personal realm to carefully examine personal knowledge related to the procedure. Rather than reflection on action or inaction, this analysis may be done prior to the procedure to inform subsequent practice. This may involve examining notes from the classroom, textbooks, ward policies and observation of practice and recording these in the journal.

Critical analysis also encourages the recognition of multiple perspectives. Very often students focus on discrepancies between their received teaching and the practice observed on the wards. In their reflection these observations can thwart their perception of their learning experience. Guided perhaps by a belief in ' perfectionism' as articulated by Watson (1999, p. 37) who suggested that nursing students are 'led to believe that only perfect practice is permissible in clinical areas'. This is not to suggest that best practice or evidence-based practice is not adhered to, but rather refers to the observation by students of expert practice as described by Benner (1999) that deviates slightly from the mechanized procedure that a student has been taught.

One such procedure may be patient hygiene. The nurse may not have attended to hygiene needs in the particular order and sequence taught to the student in the classroom and this may be a cause for concern for the student. Critical analysis of situations encourages the student to explore multiple perspectives. A non-judgemental student-led discussion after observing the procedure is required so that the student may understand the perspective of the nurse and this would be a good learning experience. There may be a very clear rationale for this deviation in procedure. It could be that the ward policy is different to that taught in the classroom. Or there may be other reasons. Whatever the justification, the idea is that the students explore the multiple facets of the situation rather than relying solely upon personal reflection and intro-spection that may be of limited value (Brechin *et al.*, 2000), particularly for junior students who often report that they don't really know what they are reflecting upon. Using the example of intramuscular injection, the student may have observed the procedure and rather than moving straight to performance under supervision it may be useful to have a discussion with the teacher or mentor to gain more insight into their perspective. In addition to elucidating any perceived discrepancies the student may learn the subtleties of expert practice as the nurse begins to articulate those aspects of prac-tice not necessarily accounted for in the procedure, such as a gentle touch of the hand during explanation.

Critical analysis also involves different levels of analysis.

This implies not only personal analysis and consideration of personal actions required in a situation, but an analysis of the context (the ward, the patient, the atmosphere, the relationships), ward policy and procedures, other people's views of the situation and the client's view. This type of analysis discourages the introspection of reflection that solely encourages the analysis of one's personal feelings in situations. The context in which interactions takes place is crucial to our understanding of events. Brechin (2000) also suggested that this analysis should be ongoing, so rather than leaving analysis as single entries in a journal they would feed into others and develop as a theme throughout the journal.

Another vehicle for the collection of such information that is gaining increasing popularity in nursing is a portfolio (Scholes *et al.*, 2004). These authors describe a portfolio as a 'purposeful collection of traditional and non-traditional work that represents a student's learning, progress and achievement over time'. Reflection commonly forms part of a portfolio, and the portfolio may be used as part components of course work assessment. The portfolio is particularly useful for outlining particular themes that can be developed. When applying a critical analysis framework the portfolio can be useful for storing the relevant information.

The next component of critical practice is critical action. Brechin (2000) suggested that one should operate with a sound skill base used with awareness of context. Having performed the necessary analysis in the first part of this cycle the student will have gained increased knowledge about the skill from analysing prior learning, ward procedures and through discussions with others. The knowledge base is already improved at the level required. It is also suggested that the student operates to question structural disadvantage, and works with difference towards empowerment that presents a challenge for students at a junior level. However it is worth reading, reflecting and observing these skills, and writing about them within the portfolio, as they are crucial to modern nursing. Contemporary notions of health and health care are based upon patient empowerment and reduction of disadvantage, so the student must begin to consider these in their practice. Using the example of the intramuscular injection, patient empowerment may simply involve providing choice as to whether a student may perform the procedure. Although it may seem pedantic, it is the beginnings of recognizing patients as equal partners in care and not passive recipients in care. After the procedure the patient's views may be elicited and this too would provide a level of patient involvement and empowerment.

The final section in the critical practice cycle is critical reflexivity. While this is the inherently personal aspect of critical practice, it involves less introspection. The student is encouraged to become engaged with practice, consider practice issues and also to negotiate understandings. Rather than the student operating from a one-sided perspective they are encouraged to share their understanding of situations and listen to the others' views to inform their view. It is also suggested that one questions one's personal values and assumptions. So that rather than operating from the 'perfectionist' stance; as articulated by Watson (1999) one is continuously questioning values and beliefs in given situations. Figure 10.2 and 10.3 are two examples of portfolio entries. Note elements of critical practice as you read.

You may have noticed that policies and current practice were taken into consideration in both entries. The use of a textbook indicated the development of a sound knowledge base. At times the writer was attempting to work towards reducing disadvantage by considering gaps in current practice. There was also an attempt towards greater patient empowerment. Ultimately critical reflexivity was present as the writer challenged their own assumptions and came to new understandings about communication practice.

Aspects of communication such as patient action, nursing action and the evolving relationship can be framed within the critical practice framework (Figure 10.4). Fundamental communication skills can be explored, developed and utilized in practice by nursing students and nurses through skills of self-awareness and reflection. This may involve experiential learning documented in diaries, journals or portfolios. Critical analysis can reveal the patient's actions and perspective and reveal the specific context for nursing action. Critical action involves empowering patients through comforting strategies,

Portfolio entry 1   Communication skills

During portfolio activity 1, I reflected upon different types of personal communication. The exploration of the communication theories and methods provided valuable additional insight into my own behaviour in this area. I was aware that I was talkative in social situations, and I considered my communication to be of satisfactory standard. The activities and reflection that I undertook during this clinical placement challenged this assumption.

This involved a critical analysis of my listening skills. It became apparent that my listening skills were poor. Whilst I often feigned this skill, in reality I let my mind wander. Such lack of engagements now strikes me as an obvious flaw. It is an essential prerequisite to attending. Clearly, its absence was a barrier to my development as a communicator.

My approach to communication in general deviated towards a person-centred approach (Sidell, 2000). However, empathy, unconditional positive regard and genuineness are crucial to this humanistic style, which in effect were absent on many occasions during that week, when I failed to listen or talked too much. I realised that in order to develop an atmosphere of trust and respect with clients or students, I needed to be a good listener. I also understood that listening is crucial to success in health education situations (see article). I became aware that reasons existed for my failure to listen (Sidell, 2000), which was mainly self-consciousness, although sometimes I just wanted to be the one doing all the talking.

During the week, I was acutely aware of daydreaming when people spoke. This new awareness, prompted by this activity, meant that I began to make a conscious effort to actually listen and attend. I found that while this took effort for the first few minutes, once I made a real effort to listen and move beyond the level basic levels of listening (Sidell, 2000), it became really easy and enjoyable.

Effective communication is a crucial component of effective nursing practice that I now aspire to. I am embarrassed to think that I have been such a poor listener and I hope that the insight that I gained from this portfolio exercise will continue to improve my listening skills and that they will become imbedded in my practice over time. This activity focused and developed personal skills that are useful to practice.

Figure 10.2   Example of portfolio entry one

styles of care and relating to patients. Critical reflexivity examines the effectiveness and development of communication through self-engagement, challenging personal assumptions and establishing the extent to which a therapeutic relationship developed and whether the communication was patient-centred.

Portfolio entry 2 Communication in Health Promotion

Learning about myself as a health promoter really took me by surprise. Rather than being merely a learning exercise, the portfolio and other activities encouraged me to review and critically assess my practice. My self-awareness grew through the exploration and justification of my own definition of health and health promotion in the portfolio. I was quite surprised that my notion of health and health promotion was firmly enshrined in the medical model of health. I considered myself already knowledgeable in this area, and I was shocked at how short sighted I had been. My practice was similar to health education (one to one and information giving) as opposed to health promotion (the total needs).

In this activity I critically reviewed and developed my ideas about my approach to health promotion. I was quite amazed to see it described as 'authoritative'. I began to understand the influences on my thinking. Local policy guided my practice. In addition the lifestyle approach, had both national and international approval (Jones, 2000a) and reflected a local response to national targets. My fellow students had a similar approach.

I thought that I had a holistic approach to nursing care as a third year student but I had not translated this holism into my personal thinking and practice in relation to health promotion. On one level, I was obviously aware of the existence of social issues, but had never considered their impact on health. I came to realise during this ward placement that health promotion should be holistic, addressing social and economic inequalities. Reflecting collective, rather than individual intervention. This learning was endorsed through discussion with my mentor.

I developed an increased understanding of the social and economic determinants of health and explored different models of health promotion (Jones 2000a). The consideration of my own beliefs about health was new to me and very enlightening. I realised that people's attitudes and actions towards health are value bound. The limits of a medical approach became apparent to me and I developed a new way of thinking about health, I became willing to move away from a lifestyle (persuasive/individualistic) approach, realizing that it was 'victim blaming'.

I began to align my thinking with changing priorities in health promotion (Jones 2000a), where health is conceptualized as a state of not just freedom from illness, but of psychological and social well-being. This latter aspect of health was illuminated in Cox et al's work (1997, cited in Jones, 2006b). This latter information astounded me. For the future, I decided that my practice would be guided by the values of the Ottawa charter social justice, participation, equity, and empowerment and reflect a less conservative and more collective approach. I was at odds with contemporary health promotion theory and practice. I realized that my approach to health promotion needed to be multi-strategy. Thus I began fundamental changes in my definitions of health and health promotion, and, the next activity, challenged the practice.

Figure 10.3 Example of portfolio entry two

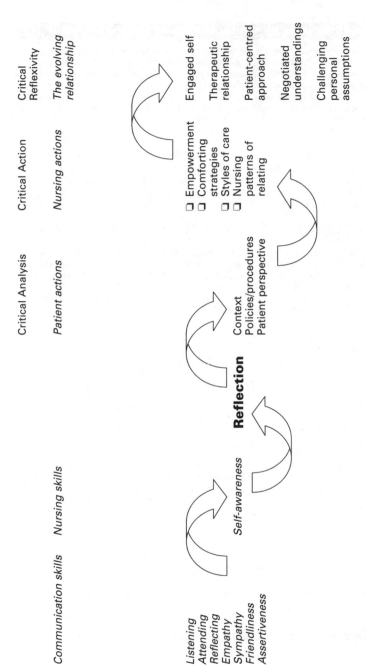

Figure 10.4 Dynamic communication model for nursing practice

Although theory and models serve to inform communication in the health care context, in a post modern era technical rationality is replaced with a more dynamic model for practice that evolves through experiential learning, critical practice and patient involvement. If the ultimate aim of nurse–patient communication is patient centredness than the conceptual models guiding care must reflect this approach too. It is no longer acceptable to continue with a narcissistic approach such as reflection. Experiential learning in the health care context requires the development of a sound knowledge base, awareness of context, inclusion of patient views, feedback from mentors and challenging of personal assumptions. All these are features of critical practice that is suggested as a way forward for development of the science of communication.

Key points

▶ An eclectic use of models is regarded as effective and useful for explaining and developing nursing practice.
▶ Methods of learning how to communicate positively and effectively with patients include the use of diaries, journals, reflection and The Critical Practice Model. This model consists of three key components, critical analysis, critical action and critical reflexivity and is regarded as a way forward for the development of the science of communication.
▶ Unlike some models of learning, experiential learning reflects the ultimate aim of nurse–patient communication, which is patient-centredness.

References

Chapter 1

Astedt-Kurki, P. and Haggman-Laitila, A. (1992) Good nursing practice as perceived by clients: A starting point for the development of professional nursing, *Journal of Advanced Nursing*, 17, 1195–9.

Attree, M. (2001) Patients' and relatives' experiences and perspectives of 'Good' and 'Not so Good' quality care, *Journal of Advanced Nursing*, 33, 456–66.

Balzer-Riley, J. (2004) *Communication in Nursing* (Missouri: Mosby).

Bateson, G. (1979) *Mind and Nature* (New York: Dutton).

Berlo, D. (1960) *The Process of Communication: An Introduction to the Theory and Practice* (New York: Holt, Rinehart & Winston).

Bradley, J.C. and Edinberg, M.A. (1990) *Communication in the Nursing Context*, 3rd edn. (Connecticut: Appleton and Lange).

DeVito, J.A. (2002) *Human Communication – The Basic Course*, 9th edn. (Massachusetts: Allyn & Bacon).

Fosbinder, D. (1994) Patient perceptions of nursing care: An emerging theory of interpersonal competence, *Journal of Advanced Nursing*, 20, 1085–93.

Hargie, O. and Dickson, D. (2004) *Skilled Interpersonal Communication: Research, Theory and Practice* (Sussex: Routledge).

Hayes, J. (1991) *Interpersonal Skills: Goal-Directed Behaviour at Work* (London: Harper Collins).

Kruijver J.P.M., Kerkstra A., Bensing J.M. and Van de Wiel H.B.M. (2001) Communication skills of nurses during interactions with simulated cancer patients, *Journal of Advanced Nursing*, 34(6), 772–9.

McCabe, C. (2004) Nurse–patient communication: An exploration of patients' experiences, *Journal of Clinical Nursing*, 13, 41–9.

McQueen, A. (2000) Nurse–patient relationships and partnership in hospital care, *Journal of Clinical Nursing*, 9, 723–31.

Miller, G.R. and Nicholson, H.E. (1976) *Communication Inquiry: A Perspective on Process* (Reading: Addison-Wesley).

Morse, J., Bottorff, J., Anderson, G., O'Brien, B. and Solberg, S. (1992) Beyond empathy: Expanding expressions of caring, *Journal of Advanced Nursing*, 17, 809–21.

Morse, J.M., De Luca Havens, G.A., and Wilson, S. (1997) The comforting interaction: Developing a model of nurse–patient relationship, *Scholarly Inquiry for Nursing Practice*, 11(4), 321–43.

Oettingen, G. and Gollwitzer, P. (2001) Goal setting and goal striving. In A. Tesser and N. Schwarz (eds), *Blackwell Handbook of Social Psychology: Intraindividual Processes* (Malden, MA: Blackwell).

Peplau, H.E. (1988) *Interpersonal Relations in Nursing* (London: MacMillan Education).

Peplau, H.E. (1952) *Interpersonal Relations in Nursing* (New York: G.P. Putnam).

Petrie, P. (1997) *Communicating with Children and Adults: Interpersonal Skills for Early Years and Play Work* (London: Arnold).

Ruesch, J. (1961) *Therapeutic Communication* (Toronto: Norton & Company Inc.).

Rosengren, K.E. (2000) *Communication: An Introduction* (London: Sage).

Sheppard, M. (1993) Client satisfaction, extended intervention and interpersonal skills in community mental health, *Journal of Advanced Nursing*, 18, 246–59.

Thorsteinsson, L.S.C.H. (2002) The quality of nursing care as perceived by individuals with chronic illnesses: The magical touch of nursing, *Journal of Clinical Nursing*, 11, 32–44.

Wilkinson, S. (199) Communication: It makes a difference, *Cancer Nursing*, 22, 17–20.

Williams, A.M. (1998) The delivery of quality nursing care: A grounded theory study of the nurse's perspective, *Journal of Advanced Nursing*, 27, 808–16.

Chapter 2

Aggleton, S.K. and Chambers, H. (2000) *Nursing Models and Nursing Practice*, 2nd edn. (Basingstoke: Macmillan Press).

Alligood, M.R. (2002) The nature of knowledge needed for nursing practice. In M.R. Alligood and A. Marriner-Tomey (eds), *Nursing Theory Utilisation and Application* (London: Mosby).

Alligood, M.R. and Marriner-Tomey, A. (2002a) Significance of theory for nursing as a discipline. In M.R. Alligood and A. Marriner-Tomey (eds), *Nursing Theorists and Their Work*, 5th edn. (London: Mosby).

Alligood, M.R. and Marriner-Tomey, A. (2002b) Introduction to nursing theory: History, terminology, and analysis is practice. In M.R. Alligood and A. Marriner-Tomey (eds), *Nursing Theorists and Their Work*, 5th edn. (London: Mosby).

Arnold, E. and Underman Boggs, K. (1999) *Interpersonal Relationships Professional Communication Skills for Nurses*, 3rd edn. (London: WB Saunders).

Berbiglia, V.A. (2002) Orem's Self-Care Deficit Nursing Theory in practice. In M.R. Alligood and A. Marriner-Tomey (eds), *Nursing Theorists and Their Work*, 5th edn. (London: Mosby).

Chambers-Evans, J., Stelling, J. and Godin, M. (1999) Learning to listen: Serendipitous outcomes of a research training experience, Journal *of Advanced Nursing*, 29 (6), 1421–6.

Costa, M.J. (2001) The lived perioperative experience of ambulatory surgery patients, *AORN Journal*, 74 (6), 874–81.

Fawcett, J. (1995) *Analysis and Evaluation of Conceptual Models of Nursing*, 3rd edn. (Philadelphia: F.A. Davies Company).

Fossum, B. and Arborelius, E. (2004) Patient-centred communication: Videotaped consultations, *Patient Education and Counseling*, 54, 163–9.

Holland, K., Jenkins, J., Solomon, J. and Whittam, S. (eds) (2004) *Applying the Roper Logan Tierney Model in Practice* (London: Churchill Livingstone).

Howard-Harwood, B. (1997) Care of the patient in the day surgical unit. In L. Markanday (ed.), *Day Surgery for Nurses* (London: Whurr).

Iggulden, H. (2004) Communicating. In K. Holland, J. Jenkins, J. Solomon and S. Whittam (eds), *Applying the Roper Logan Tierney Model in Practice*. (London: Churchill Livingstone).

Ito, M. and Lambert, V.A. (2002) Communication effectiveness of nurses working in a variety of settings within a large university teaching hospital in western Japan, *Nursing and Health Sciences*, 4, 149–53.

Jacobson, A.F. (2000) Research utilization in nursing: The power of one, *Orthopedic Nursing*, 19 (6), 61–5.

Jenner, E.A. (1998) A case study analysis of nurses' roles, education and training needs associated with patient-focused care, *Journal of Advanced Nursing*, 27, 1087–95.

Keating, D., Bellchambers, H., Bujack, E., Cholowski, K., Conway, J. and Neal, P. (2002) Communication: Principal barrier to nurse–consumer partnerships, *International Journal of Nursing Practice*, 8, 16–22.

Kim, H.S. (1983) *The Nature of Theoretical Thinking in Nursing* (Connecticut: Appleton-Century Crofts).

Martin, G. (1998) Ritual action and its effect on the role of the nurse as advocate, *Journal of Advanced Nursing*, 27, 189–94.

McKenna, H. (1997) *Nursing Theories and Models* (London: Routledge).

Michie, S., Miles, J. and Weinman, J. (2003) Patient-centredness in chronic illness: What is it and does it matter? *Patient Education and Counseling*, 51, 197–260.

Orem, D. E. (1971, 1980, 1985, 1991, 1995, 2001) *Nursing: Concepts of Practice*, 1st, 2nd, 3rd, 4th 5th and 6th edns. (London: Mosby).

Pearson, A., Vaughan, B. and Fitzgerald, M. (2000) *Nursing Models for Practice*, 2nd edn. (London: Butterworth Heinemann).

Peplau, H.E. (1952, 1991) *Interpersonal Relations in Nursing A Conceptual Frame of Reference for Psychodynamic Nursing* (New York: Springer).

Riegel, B., Tomason, T., Carlson, B. and Gocka, L. (1996) Are nurses still practicing coronary precautions? A national survey of nursing care of acute myocardial infarction patients, *American Journal of Critical Care*, 5, 91–8.

Roper, N., Logan, W.W. and Tierney, A.J. (1980, 1985, 1990, 1996) *The Elements of Nursing: A Model for Nursing Based on a Model for Living*, 1st, 2nd, 3rd and 4th edns. (London: Churchill Livingstone)

Roper, N., Logan, W.W. and Tierney, A.J. (2001) *The Roper Logan Tierney Model of Nursing Based on Activities of Living* (London: Churchill Livingstone).

Strange, F. (2001) The persistence of ritual in nursing practice, *Clinical Effectiveness in Nursing*, 5(4), 177–83.

Wissow, L.S. (2004) Communication and malpractice claims – where are we now? *Patient Education and Counseling*, 52(1), 3–5.

Chapter 3

Buber, M. (1958) *I and Thou*, 2nd edn. R.G. Smith (trans.). (New York: Scribner's).

Brooks, I. (2003) *The Chambers Dictionary* (London: Harpers Publishing).

Dworetzky, J.P. (1997) *Psychology*, 6th edn. (California: Brooks/Cole).

Gallop, R. and O'Brien, L. (2003) Re-establishing psychodynamic theory as foundational knowledge for psychiatric/mental health nursing, *Issues in Mental Health Nursing*, 24, 213–27.

Langwitz, W.A., Eich, P., Kiss, A. and Wossmer, B. (1998) Improving communication skills – a randomized controlled behaviorally oriented intervention study for residents in internal medicine, *Psycho-somatic Medicine*, 60, 268–76.

Maslow, A.H. (1954) *Motivation and Personality* (New York: Harper & Row).

McCabe, C. (2004) Nurse–patient communication: An exploration of patients' experiences, *Journal of Clinical Nursing*, 13, 41–9.

Menzies, I. (1970) *The Functioning of the Social Systems as a Defence Against Anxiety* (London: Tavistock Institute of Human Relations).

Morse, J.M., De Luca Havens, G.A. and Wilson, S. (1997) The comforting interaction: Developing a model of nurse–patient relationship, *Scholarly Inquiry for Nursing Practice*, 11(4), 321–43.

O'Kelly, G. (1998) Countertransference in the nurse–patient relationship: A review of the literature, *Journal of Advanced Nursing*, 28(2), 391–7.

Peplau, H.E. (1952) *Interpersonal Relations in Nursing* (New York: Putnam's).

Rogers, C.R. (1961) *On Becoming a Person: A Therapist's View of Psychotherapy* (Boston: Houghton Mifflin).

Rogers, C.R. (1969) *On Becoming a Person: A Therapist's View of Psychotherapy*, 2nd edn. (Boston: Houghton Mifflin).

Ruesch, J. (1973) *Therapeutic Communication* (New York: W.W. Norton & Company).

Wondrak, R. (1998) *Interpersonal Skills for Nurses and Health Care Professionals* (Oxford: Blackwell Science).

Chapter 4

Argyle, M. (1990) *Bodily Communication*, 2nd edn. (London: Routledge).

Caris-Verhallen, W.M.C.M, de Gruijter, I.M., Kerkstra, A. and Bensing, J.M. (1999) Factors related to nurse communication with elderly people, *Journal of Advanced Nursing*, 30(5), 1106–17.

Freshwater, D. (2003) *Counselling Skills for Nurses, Midwives and Health Visitors* (Maidenhead: Open University Press).

Gibbons, M.B. (1993) Listening to the lived experience of loss, *Pediatric Nursing*, 6, 597–9.

Hargie, O. and Dickson, D. (2004) *Skilled Interpersonal Communication: Research, Theory and Practice*, 4th edn. (London: Routledge).

Kunyk, D. (2001) Clarification of conceptualizations of empathy, *Journal of Advanced Nursing*, 35(3), 317–25.

McCabe, C. (2004) Nurse–patient communication: An exploration of patients' experiences, *Journal of Clinical Nursing*, 13, 41–9.

McCann, K. and McKenna, P.H. (1993) An examination of touch between nurses and elderly patients in a continuing care setting in Northern Ireland, *Journal of Advanced Nursing*, 18, 838–46.

McKay, M. Davis, M. and Fanning, P. (1995) 'Expressing'. In J. Stewart (ed.), *Bridges not walls*, 7th edn. (Boston: McGraw-Hill).

Milburn, M., Baker, M., Gardner, P., Hornsby, R. and Rogers, L. (1995) Nursing care that patients value, *British Journal of Nursing*, 4(18), 1094–8.

Morse, J.M., Bottorff, J., Anderson, G., O'Brien, B. and Solberg, S. (1992) Beyond Empathy: Expanding expressions of caring, Journal *of Advanced Nursing*, 17, 809–21.

Peplau H.E. (1997) Peplau's Theory of Interpersonal Relations, *Nursing Science Quarterly*, 10(4), 162–7.

Perry B. (1996) Influence of nurse gender on the use of silence, touch and humour, *International Journal of Palliative Nursing*, 7, 7–14.

Reynolds W. and Scott P.A. (2000) Nursing, empathy and perception of the moral, *Journal of Advanced Nursing*, 32(1), 235–42.

Routasalo P. (1999) Physical touch in nursing studies: A literature review, Journal *of Advanced Nursing*, 30(4), 843–50.

Williams, A. (2001) A study of practicing nurses' perceptions and experiences of intimacy within the nurse–patient relationship, *Journal of Advanced Nursing*, 32(2), 188–96.

Wiseman T. (1996) A concept analysis of empathy, *Journal of Advanced Nursing*, 23(6), 1162–7.

Wondrak R. (1998) *Interpersonal Skills for Nurses and Health Care Professionals* (Oxford: Blackwell Science).

Chapter 5

Aggleton, P. and Chalmers, H. (2000) *Nursing Models and Nursing Practice*, 2nd edn. (Basingstoke: Palgrave).

Arnold, E. and Underman Boggs, K. (1999) *Interpersonal Relationships Professional Communication Skills for Nurses*, 3rd edn. (London: W.B. Saunders Company).

Bergen, A. (1992) Evaluating nursing care of the terminally ill in the community: A case study approach, *International Journal of Nursing Studies*, 31, 499–510.

Betts, A. (2003) Improving communication. In R.B. Ellis, B. Gates, and N. Kenworthy (eds), *Interpersonal Communication in Nursing Theory and Practice*, 2nd edn. (London: Churchill Livingstone) 73–85.

Booth K., Maguire P.M. and Butterworth T. (1996) Perceived professional support and the use of blocking behaviours by hospice nurses, *Journal of Advanced Nursing*, 24, 522–7.

Bowler, I.M.W. (1993) Stereotypes of women of Asian descent in midwifery: Some evidence, *Midwifery*, 9(1), 7–16.

Buber, M. (1958) *I and Thou*, 2nd ed, R.G. Smith (trans.) (New York: Scribner's).

Burnard, P. (1997) *Effective Communication Skills for Health Professionals*, 2nd edn. (Cheltenham: Nelson Thornes).

Chambers-Evans, J., Stelling, J. and Godin, M. (1999) Learning to listen: Serendipitous outcomes of a research training experience, *Journal of Advanced Nursing*, 29(6), 1421–6.

Corbett, T. (2001) The nurse as a professional carer. In R.B. Ellis, R.J. Gates and N. Kenworthy (eds), *Interpersonal Communication in Nursing Theory and Practice* (London: Churchill Livingstone).

Costa, M.J. (2001) The lived perioperative experience of ambulatory surgery patients, *AORN Journal*, 74(6), 874–81.

Cree, V.E., Kay, H., Tisdall, K. and Wallace, J. (2004) Stigma and parental HIV, *Qualitative Social Work*, 3(1), 7–25.

Crotty, M. (1985) Communication between nurses and their patients, *Nurse Education Today*, 2, 130–4.

Davies, M.M. and Bath, P.A. (2001) The maternity information concerns of Somali women in the United Kingdom, *Journal of Advanced Nursing*, 36(2), 237–45.

DeVos, J. (1989) The patient with brain dysfunction. In S. Lewis, R. Dailey Knowles Grainger, W.A. McDowell, R.J. Gregory and R.L. Messner (eds), *Manual of Psychosocial Nursing Interventions Promoting Mental Health in Medical-Surgical Settings* (London: W.B. Saunders Company), 65–86.

Doak, C.C., Doak, L.G. and Root, J.H. (1985) *Teaching Patients With Low Literacy Skill* (Philadelphia: J.B. Lippincott).

Driscoll, A. (2000) Managing post-discharge care at home: An analysis of patients' and their carers' perceptions of information received during their stay in hospital, *Journal of Advanced Nursing*, 31(5), 1165–73.

Dworetzky, J.P. (1997) *Psychology*, 6th edn. (California: Brooks/Cole Publishing Company).

Edwards, S.C. (1998) An anthropological interpretation of nurses' and patients' perceptions of the use of space and touch, *Journal of Advanced Nursing*, 28(4), 809–17.

Edwards, A., Evans, R. and Elwyn, G. (2003) Manufactured but not imported: New directions for research in shared decision making support and skills, *Patient Education and Counseling*, 50(1), 33–8.

Fossum, B. and Arborelius, E. (2004) Patient-centred communication: Videotaped consultations, *Patient Education and Counseling*, 54, 163–9.

Foster, J.H. and Onyeukwu, C. (2003) The attitudes of forensic nurses to substance using service users, *Journal of Psychiatric and Mental Health Nursing*, 10(5), 578–84.

Gallant, M.H., Beaulieu, M.C. and Carnveale, F.A. (2002) Partnership: An analysis of the concept within the nurse–client relationship, *Journal of Advanced Nursing*, 40(2), 149–57.

Gallop, R. and O'Brien, L. (2003) Re-establishing psychodynamic theory as foundational knowledge for psychiatric/mental health nursing, *Issues in Mental Health Nursing*, 24, 213–27.

Gibbons, M.B. (1993) Listening to the lived experience of loss, *Pediatric Nursing*, 6, 597–9.

Gleeson, M. and Timmins, F. (2004) The use of touch to enhance the nursing care of older clients in long-term mental health care facilities, *Journal of Psychiatric and Mental Health Nursing*, 11, 514–45.

Green, J.M., Kitzinger, J.V. and Coupland, V.A. (1990) Stereotypes of childbearing women: A look at some evidence, *Midwifery*, 6(3), 125–32.

Haggman-Laitila A. and Astedt-Kurki P. (1994) What is expected of the nurse–client interaction and how these expectations are realized in Finnish health care, *International Journal of Nursing Studies*, 31, 253–61.

Hindle, S.A. (2003) Psychological factors affecting communication. In R.B. Ellis, B. Gates and N. Kenworthy (eds), *Interpersonal Communication in Nursing Theory and Practice*, 2nd edn. (London: Churchill Livingstone) 53–71.

Hodges, V., Sanford, D. and Elzinga, R. (1986) The role of ward structure on nursing staff behaviours: An observational study of three psychiatric wards, *Acta Psychiatrica Scandinavica*, 73, 6–11.

Hollinger, L.M. and Buschmann, M.B.T. (1993) Factors influencing the perception of touch by elderly nursing home residents and their health care givers, *International Journal of Nursing Studies*, 30(5), 445–61.

Hostutler J.J., Taft S.H. and Snyder C. (1999) Patient needs in the Emergency Department: Nurses' and patients' perceptions, *Journal of Nursing Administration*, 29, 433–50.

Howard-Harwood, B. (1997) Care of the patient in the day surgical unit. In L. Markanday (ed.), *Day Surgery for Nurses* (London: Whurr).

Ito, M. and Lambert, V.A. (2002) Communication effectiveness of nurses working in a variety of settings within a large university teaching hospital in western Japan *Nursing and Health Sciences*, 4, 149–53.

Jacobson, A.F. (2000) Research utilization in nursing: The power of one, *Orthopedic Nursing*, 19(6), 61–5.

James, D. (2000) Patients perceptions of day surgery, *British Journal of Perioperative Nursing*, 10(9), 466–72.

Jarman, F. (1995) Communication problems: A patient's view, *Nursing Times*, 91, 30–1.

Jarrett N.J. and Payne S.A. (2000) Creating and maintaining 'optimism' in cancer care communication, *International Journal of Nursing Studies*, 37, 81–90.

Jorm, A.F., Korten, A.E., Jacomb, P.A., Christensen, H. and Henderson, S. (1999) Attitudes toward people with a mental disorder: A survey of the Australian public and health professionals, *Australian and New Zealand Journal of Psychiatry*, 33, 77–83.

Keating, D., Bellchambers, H., Bujack, E., Cholowski, K., Conway, J. and Neal, P. (2002) Communication: Principal barrier to nurse–consumer partnerships, *International Journal of Nursing Practice*, 8, 16–22.

Kirkham, M., Stapleton, H., Curtis, P. and Thomas, G. (2002) Stereotyping as a professional defence mechanism, *British Journal of Midwifery*, 10(9), 549–52.

McCabe, C. (2004) Nurse–patient communication: An exploration of patients' experiences, *Journal of Clinical Nursing*, 13, 41–9.

McCann, K. and McKenna, H. (1993) An examination of touch between nurses and elderly patients in a continuing care setting in Northern Ireland, *Journal of Advanced Nursing*, 18, 838–46.

Markanday, L. (ed.) (1997) *Day Surgery for Nurses* (London: Whurr).

Martin, G. (1998) Ritual action and its effect on the role of the nurse as advocate, *Journal of Advanced Nursing*, 27, 189–94.

Maslow, A.H. (1954) *Motivation and personality* (New York: Harper & Row).

Mavundla, T.R. and Uys, LR. (1997) The attitudes of nurses toward mentally ill people in a general hospital setting in Durban, *Curationis*, 20(2), 3–7.

Michie, S., Miles, J. and Weinman, J. (2003) Patient-centredness in chronic illness: What is it and does it matter? *Patient Education and Counseling*, 51, 197–260.

Mitchell, M. (1997) Patients' perceptions of pre-operative preparation for day surgery, *Journal of Advanced Nursing*, 26(2), 356–63.

Morrall, P. (2003) Social factors affecting communication. In R.B. Ellis, R.J. Gates and N. Kenworthy (eds), *Interpersonal Communication in Nursing Theory and Practice*, 2nd edn. (London: Churchill Livingstone) 33–51.

Nesbitt Blondis, M. and Jackson, B.E. (1982) *Nonverbal Communication with Patients, Back to the Human Touch*, 2nd edn. (New York: John Wiley & Sons).

Northouse, L.L. and Northouse, P.G. (1998) *Health Communication Strategies for Health Professionals*, 3rd edn. (London: Prentice Hall International).

O'Brien, L. (2000) Nurse–client relationships: The experience of community psychiatric nurses, *Australian and New Zealand Journal of Mental Health Nursing*, 9(4), 184–94.

O'Kelly, G. (1998) Countertransference in the nurse–patient relationship: A review of the literature, *Journal of Advanced Nursing*, 28(2), 391–7.

O' Shea, J. (2004) Parents experience of neonatal ICU 5th Annual Research Conference, 3–5 November 2004. (Dublin: School of Nursing and Midwifery, University of Dublin, Trinity College Unpublished proceedings).

Ogden, J. (2000) *Health Psychology A Textbook*, 2nd edn. (Buckingham: Open University Press).

Oliver, S. and Redfern, S.J. (1991) Interpersonal communication between nurses and elderly patients: Refinement of an observation schedule, *Journal of Advanced Nursing*, 16, 30–38.

Orem, D.E. (2001) *Nursing: Concepts of Practice*, 6th edn. (London: Mosby).

Otte, D. (1996) Patients' perspectives and experiences of day surgery, *Journal of Advanced Nursing*, 23(6), 1228–37.

Pearson, A, Vaughan, B. and Fitzgerald M. (2000) *Nursing Models for Practice*, 2nd edn. (London: Butterworth Heinemann).

Peplau, H.E. (1952, 1991) *Interpersonal Relations in Nursing: A Conceptual Frame of Reference for Psychodynamic Nursing* (New York: Springer).

Phillips, J. (1992) Breaking down the barriers, *Nursing Times*, 88(35), 30–1.

Reid, N.G. (1985) *Wards in Chancery? Nurse Training in the Clinical Area* (London: Royal College of Nursing).

Riegel, B., Tomason, T., Carlson, B. and Gocka, L. (1996) Are nurses still practicing coronary precautions? A national survey of nursing care of acute myocardial infarction patients, *American Journal of Critical Care*, 5, 91–8.

Rogan Foy, C. and Timmins, F. (2004) Improving communication in day surgery settings, *Nursing Standard*, 17(9), 37–43.

Rogers, C.R. (1961) *On Becoming a Person* (Houghton Mifftin, Boston).

Röndahl, G., Innala, S. and Carlsson, M. (2004) Nursing staff and nursing students' emotions towards homosexual patients and their wish to refrain from nursing, if the option existed, *Scandinavian Journal of Caring Sciences*, 18(1), 19–26.

Roper, N., Logan, W.W. and Tierney, A.J. (2001) *The Roper Logan Tierney Model of Nursing Based on Activities of Living* (London: Churchill Livingstone).

Routasalo, P. (1996) Non-necessary touch in the nursing care of elderly people, *Journal of Advanced Nursing*, 23(5), 904–11.

Sidell, M. (2000) Supporting individuals and facilitating change: The role of counseling skills. In J. Katz, A. Perberdy and J. Douglas (eds), *Promoting Health: Knowledge and Practice* (Basingstoke: Palgrave), 140–61.

Simons, J. and Robertson, E. (2002) Poor communication and knowledge deficits: Obstacles to effective management of children's postoperative pain, *Journal of Advanced Nursing*, 40(1), 78–86.

Stein-Parbury, J. (1993) *Patient and Person: Developing Interpersonal Skills in Nursing* (Melbourne: Churchill Livingstone).

Strange, F. (2001) The persistence of ritual in nursing practice, *Clinical Effectiveness in Nursing*, 5(4), 177–83.

Tierney, A.J. (1998) Nursing models: extant or extinct? *Journal of Advanced Nursing*, 8(1), 77–85.

Thomas, V. and Dines, A. (1994) The health care needs of ethnic minority groups: Are nurses and individuals playing their part? *Journal of Advanced Nursing*, 20(5), 802–8.

Valimaki, M., Suominen, T. and Peate, I. (1998) Attitudes of professionals, students and general public to HIV/AIDS and people with HIV/AIDS: A review of the research, *Journal of Advanced Nursing*, 27(4), 752–9.

Williams, K., Kemper, S. and Hummert, L. (2004) Enhancing communication with older adults: Overcoming elderspeak, *Journal of Gerontological Nursing*, 30(10), 17–25.

Wondrak, R. (1998) *Interpersonal Skills for Nurses and Health Care Professionals* (Oxford: Blackwell Science).

Wood, A.F. and Alligood, M.R. (2002) Nursing: Normal science for nursing practice. In M.R. Alligood and A. Marriner-Tomey (eds), *Nursing Theory Utilisation and Application* (London: Mosby).

Zion, A.B. and Aiman, J. (1989) Level of reading difficulty in American College of Obstetrics and Gynaecology patient education pamphlets, *Obstetrics and Gynaecology*, 74(6), 955–60.

Chapter 6

Anonymous (1994) Cot death – A mothers story, *New World of Irish Nursing*, 2(1), 10–12.

Craib, I. (1999) Reflections on mourning in the modern world, *International Journal of Palliative Nursing*, 5(2), 87–9.

Engel, G.L. (1972) Grief and grieving. In L. Schwartz and S. Schwartz (eds), *The Psychodynamics of Patient Care* (New York: Prentice Hall).

Giger, J.N. and Davidhizar, R.E. (1999) *Transcultural Nursing: Assessment and Intervention*, 3rd edn. (St. Louis: Mosby).

Grypma, S. (1993) Culture shock, *The Canadian Nurse*, Sept., 33–6.

Jones, D.C. and Van Amelsvoort-Jones, G.M.M. (1986) Communication patterns between nursing staff and the ethnic elderly in a long term care facility, *Journal of Advanced Nursing*, 11(3), 265–72.

Kreigh, H. and Perko, J. (1983) *Psychiatric and Mental Health Nursing: A Commitment to Care and Concern*, 2nd edn. (Reston, VA: Reston Publishing Company).

Kubler-Ross, E. (1973) *On Death and Dying* (London: Tavistock).

Lea, A. (1994) Nursing in today's multicultural society: A transcultural perspective, *Journal of Advanced Nursing*, 20, 307–13.

Leininger, M. (1991) Transcultural nursing: The study and practice field, *Imprint*, 38(2), 55–66.

Lindemann, E. (1994) Symptomatology and management of acute grief, *American Journal of Psychiatry*, 101, 141–8.

Stockwell, F. (1972) *The Unpopular Patient* (London: Royal College of Nursing).

Windsor-Richards, K. and Gillies, P.A. (1988) Racial grouping and women's experiences of giving birth in hospital, *Midwifery*, 4, 171–6.

Woollett, A. and Dosanjh-Matwala, N. (1990) Postnatal care: The attitudes and experiences of Asian women in East London, *Midwifery*, 6(4), 178–84.

Chapter 7

Alberti, R.E. and Emmons, M.E. (1986) *Your Perfect Right: A Guide to Assertive Behaviour*, 4th edn. (St. Lois Obispo: Impact Publishers).

Arnold E. (2003) Developing therapeutic communication skills in the nurse–client relationship. In E. Arnold and K. Underman Boggs (eds), *Interpersonal Relationships: Professional Communication Skills for Nurses*, 4th edn. (St. Louis, MO: Saunders).

Aschenbrener, C.A. and Siders, C.T. (1999) Conflict management. Managing low-to-mid intensity conflict in the health care setting, Part 2, *Physician Executive*, 25(5), 44–50.

Baker, K.M. (1995) Improving staff nurse conflict resolution skills, *Nursing Economics*, 13(5), 295–8.

Balzer Riley, J. (2000) *Communication in Nursing*, 4th edn. (St. Louis: Mosby).

Brechin, A. (2000) Introducing critical practice. In A. Brechin, H. Brown and M. Eby (eds), *Critical Practice in Health and Social Care* (London: Sage Publications) 25–47.

Domon, Y. (1997) The effect of personal relationships on nursing professional autonomy in the work environment, *Journal of St. Luke's Society for Nursing Research*, 1(1), 45–51.

Dowling, S., Martin, R., Skidmore, P., Doyal, L., Cameron, A. and Lloyd, S. (2000) Nurses taking on junior doctors work: A confusion of accountability. In C. Davies, L. Finlay and A. Bullman (eds), *Changing Practice in Health and Social Care* (London, Sage Publications).

Farrell, G.A. (2001) From tall poppies to squashed weeds: Why don't nurses pull together more? *Journal of Advanced Nursing*, 35(1), 26–33.

Gregory Dawes, G.S. (1999) Harnessing energy to overcome conflict, *Association of Operating Room Nurses AORN Journal*, 70(4), 562–5.

McCabe, C. and Timmins, F. (2003) Teaching assertiveness to undergraduate nursing students, *Nurse Education in Practice*, 3(1), 30–42.

McCartan, P. (2001) The identification and analysis of assertive behaviours in nurses. Unpublished PhD Thesis (University of Ulster: School of Nursing and Midwifery).

McElhaney, R. (1996) Conflict management in nursing administration, *Nursing Management*, 27(3), 49–50.

Percival, J. (2001) Don't be too nice, *Nursing Standard*, 15(19), 22.

Poroch, D. and McIntosh, W. (1995) Barriers to assertive skills in nurses, *Australian and New Zealand Journal of Mental Health Nursing*, 4, 113–23.

Porritt, L. (1990) *Interaction Strategies. An Introduction for Health Professionals*, 2nd edn. (Melbourne: Churchill Livingstone).

Rakos, R.F. (2003) Asserting and confronting. In O.D.W. Hargie (ed.), *The Handbook of Communication Skills*, 2nd edn. (London: Routledge).

Saks, M. (2000) Professionalism and health care. In C. Davies, L. Finlay and A. Bullman (eds), *Changing Practice in Health and Social Care*, (London: Sage Publications).

Schroeder, H.E., Rakos, R.F. and Moe, J. (1983) The social perception of assertive behaviour as a function of response class and gender, *Behaviour Therapy*, 14, 534–44.

Taylor, B. (1989) *Assertiveness and the Management of Conflict: Including Supplementary Trainer's Workshop Notes* (Leeds: Beechwood Conference Centre).

Timmins, F. and McCabe, L. (2005) Nurses' and midwives' assertive behaviour in the workplace, *Journal of Advanced Nursing*, 51(1), 38–45.

Underman Boggs, K. (2003) Resolving conflict between nurse and client. In E. Arnold and K. Underman Boggs (eds), *Interpersonal Relationships: Professional Communication Skills for Nurses*, 4th edn. (St. Louis, MO: Saunders).

Valentine, P.E.B. (1995) Management of conflict: Do nurses/women handle it differently? *Journal of Advanced Nursing*, 22, 142–9.

Valentine, P.E.B. (2001) A gender perspective on conflict management strategies of nurses, *Journal of Nursing Scholarship*, 33(1), 69–74.

Willis, L. and Daisley, J. (1994) *Springboard Women's Developmental Workbook* (Stroud: Hawthorne Press).

Willis, L. and Daisley, J. (1995) *The Assertive Trainer: A Practical Handbook for Trainers and Running Assertiveness Courses* (Maidenhead: McGraw-Hill).

Chapter 8

Blackwells Dictionary of Nursing (Oxford: Blackwell Scientific Publication, 1994).

Colyer, H.M. (2004) The construction and development of health professions: Where will it end? *Journal of Advanced Nursing*, 48(4), 406–12.

Dimond, B. (1999) *Patients' Rights, Responsibilities and the Nurse*, 2nd edn. (Wiltshire: Quay Books).

English Dictionary for Students (Teddington: Peter Collins Publishers Ltd).

Gadow, S. (1989) Clinical subjectivity – advocacy for silent patients, *Nursing Clinics of North America*, 24(2), 535–41.

Gates, B. (1994) *Advocacy: A Nurses' Guide* (London: Scutari Press).

Hancock, H. (1997) Professional responsibility: Implications for nursing practice within the realms of cardiothoracics, *Journal of Advanced Nursing*, 25, 1054–60.

Hart, C. (2004) *Nurses and Politics; The Impact of Power and Practice* (London: Palgrave Macmillan).

Henderson, V. (1996) *The Nature of Nursing: A Definition and its Implications for Practice, Research, and Education* (New York: Macmillan).

Hewitt, J. (2002) A critical review of the arguments debating the role of the nurse advocate, *Journal of Advanced Nursing*, 37(5), 439–45.

Kelly, B. (1998) Preserving moral integrity: A follow up study with new graduate nurses, *Journal of Advanced Nursing*, 28(5), 1134–45.

Krebs, L.U., Myers, J., Decker, G., Kinzler, J., Asfahani, P. and Jackson, J. (1996) The oncology nursing image: Lifting the mist, *Oncology Nursing Forum*, 23, 1297–304.

Liaschenko, J. and Peter, E. (2004) Nursing ethics and conceptualisations of nursing: Profession, practice and work, *Journal of Advanced Nursing*, 46(5), 488–95.

Llewellyn, P. (2004) Nursing and advocacy in person centred planning, *Learning Disability Practice*, 7(9), 14–17.

Mallik, M. and McHale, J. (1995) Support for advocacy, *Nursing Times*, 25(91), 28–30.

Peter, E., Lunardi, V.L. and Macfarlane, A. (2004) Nursing resistance as ethical action: Literature review, *Journal of Advanced Nursing*, 46(4), 403–16.

Redman, B.K. and Fry, S.T. (2000) Nurses' ethical conflicts: What is really known about them? *Nursing Ethics*, 7(4), 360–6.

Rogers, C.R. (1961) *On Becoming a Person* (Boston: Houghton Mifftin).

Rutty, J.E. (1998) The nature of philosophy of science, theory and knowledge relating to nursing and professionalism, *Journal of Advanced Nursing*, 28(2), 243–50.

Takase, M., Kershaw, E. and Burt, L. (2001) Nurse–environment misfit and nursing practice, *Journal of Advanced Nursing*, 35(6), 819–26.

Tschudin, V. (2003) *Ethics in Nursing: The Caring Relationship*, 3rd edn. (London: Butterworth Heinemann).

Walsh, M. (2000) *Nursing Frontiers: Accountability and the Boundaries of Care* (Oxford: Butterworth-Heinemann).

Wilson, J. (1998) Clinical governance, *British Journal of Nursing*, 7(16), 985–6.

Chapter 9

Astedt-Kurki, P. and Haggman-Laitila, A. (1992) Good nursing practice as perceived by clients: A starting point for the development of professional nursing, *Journal of Advanced Nursing*, 17(10), 1195–9.

Bandura, A. (1977) *Self-efficacy: The Exercise of Control* (New York: Freeman).

Bandura, A. (1986) *Social Foundations of Thought and Action: A Social Cognitive Theory* (Englewood Cliffs, NJ: Prentice Hall).

Bandura, A. (2000) Cultivate self-efficacy for personal and organizational effectiveness. In E.A. Locke (ed.), *Handbook of Principles of Organization Behavior* (Oxford: Blackwell), 120–36.

Barnett, R. (1997) *Higher Education: A Critical Business* (Buckingham: SRHE and Open University Press).

Betts, A. (2003) Improving communication. In R.B. Ellis, B. Gates and N. Kenworthy (eds), *Interpersonal Communication in Nursing Theory and Practice*, 2nd edn. (London: Churchill Livingstone), 73–83.

Brechin, A., Brown, H. and Eby, M. (eds) (2000) *Critical Practice in Health and Social Care* (London: Sage Publications).

Brechin, A. (2000) Introducing critical practice. In A. Brechin, H. Brown and M. Eby (eds), *Critical Practice in Health and Social Care* (London: Sage Publications), 25–47.

Burnard, P. (1985) *Learning Human Skills* (London: Heinmann).

Burnard, P. (1992) *Know Yourself! Self-Awareness Actitivities for Nurses and Other Health Professionals* (London: Scutari Press).

Burnard, P. (1997) *Know Yourself! Self-Awareness Activities for Nurses and Other Health Professionals*, 2nd edn. (London: Whurr).

Burns, S. and Bulman, C. (2000) *Reflective Practice in Nursing: the Growth of The Professional Practitioner* 2nd edn. (Oxford, Blackwell Science).

Carroll, M., Curtis, L., Higgins, A., Nicholl, H., Redmond, R. and Timmins, F. (2002) Is there a place for reflective practice in the nursing curriculum? *Clinical Effectiveness in Nursing*, 6(1), 36–41.

Chapman, A. (2005) *Business Balls Free Organisational and Personal Development*, online at www.businessballs.com (accessed 16 May 2005).

Davidhizar, R. (1993) Self-confidence: A requirement for collaborative practice, *Dimensions of Critical Care Nursing*, 12, 218–22.

Dewey, J. (1933) *How We Think* (Boston: Heath & Co.).

Ellis, R. and Gates, B. (2003) The person in communication. In R.B. Ellis, B. Gates and N. Kenworthy (eds), *Interpersonal Communication in Nursing Theory and Practice*, 2nd edn. (London: Churchill Livingstone) 17–31.

Gibbs, G. (1988) *Learning by Doing: A Guide to Teaching and Learning Methods* (Oxford: Further Education Unit).

Government of Ireland (2000) *A Strategy for Pre-Nursing Education Nursing Education Degree Programme* (Dublin, The Stationery Office).

Grainger, R.D. (1990) Self-confidence: A feeling you can create, *American Journal of Nursing*, 90(10), 12.

Hannigan, B. (2001) A discussion of the strengths and weaknesses of 'reflection' in nursing practice and education, *Journal of Clinical Nursing*, 10(2), 278–83.

Jensen, S.K. and Joy, C. (2005) Exploring a model to evaluate levels of reflection in baccalaureate nursing students' journals, *Journal of Nursing Education*, 44(3), 139–44.

Johns, C. (1999) Reflection as empowerment? *Nursing Inquiry*, 6(4), 241–6.

Kantcheva, D.A. and Eckroth-Bucher, M. (2002) Self-awareness in psychiatric nursing. . . . Philosophical basis and practice of self-awareness in psychiatric nursing, *Journal of Psychosocial Nursing and Mental Health Services*, 39(2), 32–9.

Luft, J. (1969) *Of Human Interaction* (Palo Alto, CA, National Press).

Mabe Newman, A. (2003) Self-concept in the nurse–client relationship. In Arnold, E. and Underman Boggs, K. (eds), *Interpersonal Relationships: Professional Communication Skills for Nurses*, 4th edn. (St. Louis, MO: Saunders).

Morse, J.M., De Luca Havens, G.A., and Wilson, S. (1997) The comforting interaction: Developing a model of nurse–patient relationship, *Scholarly Inquiry for Nursing Practice*, 1(4), 321–43.

Newell, R. (2002) Is there a place for reflection in the nursing curriculum? (editorial), *Clinical Effectiveness in Nursing*, 6(1), 42–3.

NHS Modernization Agency Leadership Centre, online at: www.executive.modern.nhs.uk/framework/personalqualities/selfawareness.aspx (accessed 16 May 2005).

O'Shea, J. (2004) Parents' experiences of the neonatal intensive care unit 5th Annual Research Conference, 3–5 November 2004 (Dublin: School of Nursing and Midwifery, University of Dublin, Trinity College).

Orem, D.E. (2001) *Nursing: Concepts of Practice*, 6th edn. (London: Mosby).

Pajares, F. (1997) Current directions in self-efficacy research, *Advances in Motivation and Achievement*, 10, 1–49.

Pearsall, J. and Trumble, B. (eds) (1996) *The Oxford English Reference Dictionary*, 2nd edn. (Oxford: Oxford University Press).

Pearson, A., Vaughan, B. and Fitzgerald, M. (2000) *Nursing Models for Practice*, 2nd edn. (London: Butterworth Heinemann).

Peplau, H.E. (1991) *Interpersonal Relations in Nursing: A Conceptual Frame of Reference for Psychodynamic Nursing* (New York: Springer).

Pinkery, S, (2000) Anti-oppressive theory and practice in social work'. In C. Davies, L. Finlay and A. Bullman (eds), *Changing Practice in Health and Social Care* (London: Sage Publications).

Queendom.com (2005) Tests, tests, tests, online at: http://www.queendom.com/tests/index.html (accessed 16 May 2005).

Rogers, C.R. (1961) *On Becoming a Person* (Boston: Houghton Mifftin).

Rowe, J. (1999) Self-awareness: Improving nurse–client interactions, *Nursing Standard*, 14(8), 37–41.

Scholz, U., Gutiérrez-Doña, B., Sud, S. and Schwarzer, R. (2002) Is perceived self-efficacy a universal construct? Psychometric findings from 25 countries, *European Journal of Psychological Assessment*, 18(3), 242–51.

Schön, D. (1983) *The Reflective Practitioner: How Professionals Think in Action* (London: Temple Smith).

Schwarzer, R. and Schmitz, G.S. (2004) Perceived self-efficacy and teacher burnout: A longitudinal study in ten schools, paper presented at the 3rd International Biennial SELF Research Conference: *Self-Concept, Motivation and Identity: Where to from here?* online at: http://self.uws.edu.au/ Conferences/2004_Schwarzer_Schmitz.pdf (accessed 24 November 2005).

Siciliano, E. (2005) *Emotions in the Workplace:Part Two: Principles for Leaders Dallas ASTD* (American Society for Training and Development) online at: http://www.dallasastd.org/news/ ASTD/Articles/emotion2.htm (accessed 16 May 2005).

Timmins, F., Mc Cabe, C., Griffiths, C. Gleeson, M. and O'Shea, J. (2005) *Lessons from Practice – Reflection on Communication across the Disciplines,* Symposium Presentation (UK: Royal College of Nursing of the United Kingdom Research Society Annual International Nursing Research Conference 9–11 March, Europa Hotel Belfast).

United Kingdom Central Council for Nursing Midwifery and Health Visiting Fitness for Practice (London: The UKCC Commission for Nursing and Midwifery Education, 1999).

Williams, A.M. (1998) The delivery of quality nursing care: A grounded theory study of the nurse's perspective, *Journal of Advanced Nursing,* 27, 808–16.

Chapter 10

Barnett, R. (1997) *Higher Education: A Critical Business* (Buckingham: SRHE and Open University Press).

Benner, P. (1924) *From Novice to Expert: Excellence and Power in Clinical Nursing Practice* (London Addison-Wesley).

Benner, P., Hooper-Kyriakidis, P. and Stannard, D. (1999) *Clinical Wisdom and Interventions in Critical Care. A Thinking in Action Approach* (London: W.B. Saunders).

Bradley, J.C. and Edinberg, M.A. (1990) *Communication in the Nursing Context,* 3rd edn. (Connecticut: Appleton and Lange).

Brechin, A., Brown, H. and Eby. M. (eds) (2000) *Critical Practice in Health and Social Care* (London: Sage Publications).

Fosbinder, D. (1994) Patient perceptions of nursing care: An emerging theory of interpersonal competence, *Journal of Advanced Nursing,* 20, 1085–93.

Gibbs, G., Palmer, A., Burns, S. and Bulman, C. (1994) *Reflective Practice in Nursing* (Oxford: Blackwell Scientific Publications).

Graeme, A. (2000) A post-modern nursing model, *Nursing Standard*, 14(34), 40–2.

Jones, L. (2000a) Promoting health: Everybody's business? In J. Katz, A. Perberdy and J. Douglas (eds). *Promoting Health: Knowledge and Practice* (Basingstoke: Palgrave), 2–17.

Jones, L. (2000b) What is health? In J. Katz, A. Perberdy and J. Douglas (eds), *Promoting Health: Knowledge and Practice* (Basingstoke: Palgrave) 18–36.

Kruijver, J.P.M., Kerkstra, A., Bensing, J.M. and Van de Wiel, H.B.M. (2001) Communication skills of nurses during interactions with simulated cancer patients, *Journal of Advanced Nursing*, 34(6), 772–9.

Lister, P. (1997) The art of nursing in a 'postmodern' context, *Journal of Advanced Nursing*, 25, 38–44.

McCabe, C. (2004) Nurse–patient communication: An exploration of patients' experiences, *Journal of Clinical Nursing*, 13, 41–9.

Marks-Maran, D. (1999) Reconstructing nursing: Evidence, artistry and the curriculum, *Nurse Education Today*, 19(1), 3–11.

Mitchell, D.P. (1996) Postmodernism, health and illness, *Journal of Advanced Nursing*, 23, 201–5.

Morse, J., Bottorff, J., Anderson, G., O'Brien, B. and Solberg, S. (1992) Beyond empathy: Expanding expressions of caring, *Journal of Advanced Nursing*, 17, 809–21.

Morse, J.M., De Luca Havens, G.A., and Wilson, S. (1997) The comforting interaction: Developing a model of nurse–patient relationship, *Scholarly Inquiry for Nursing Practice*, 11(4), 321–43.

Parton, N. (1994) Problematics of government post modernity and social work, *British Journal of Social Work*, 24(1), 9–32.

Reed, P.G. (1995) A treatise on nursing knowledge development for the 21st century: Beyond postmodernism, *Advances in Nursing Science*, 17(3), 70–84.

Scholes, J., Webb, C., Gray, M., Endacott, R., Miller, C., Jasper, M. and McMullan, M. (2004) Making portfolios work in practice, *Journal of Advanced Nursing*, 46(6), 595–603.

Sidell, M. (2000) Supporting individuals and facilitating change: The role of counseling skills. In J. Katz, A. Perberdy and J. Douglas (eds), *Promoting Health: Knowledge and Practice* (Basingstoke: Palgrave, 140–60.

Spitzer, A. (1998a) Nursing in the health care system of the postmodern world: Crossroads, paradoxes and complexity, *Journal of Advanced Nursing*, 28(1), 164–71.

Spitzer, A. (1998b) Moving into the information era: Does the current nursing paradigm still hold? *Journal of Advanced Nursing*, 28(4), 786–93.

Timmins, F. (2002) Critical care nursing in the 21st century, *Intensive and Critical Care Nursing Journal*, 18, 118–27.

Watson, J. (1999) *Post-Modern Nursing and Beyond* (London: Churchill Livingstone).

Watson, J. (2005) Watson's Caring Science, online at: http://www2.uchsc.edu/son/caring/content/Definition.asp accessed 27 May 2005.

Index